Healed From Lyme

Natural Treatments

That Nourish The Immune System

And Heal The Body

Tom Pote

Medical Disclaimer

The information in this book is not intended to replace the advice of a physician or other medical professional. This book is intended for informational purposes. Readers of this book are solely responsible for their own healthcare decisions. The author and publisher of this book do not accept responsibility for any adverse effects individuals may claim to experience directly or indirectly from this book. Any references to other people's work, books or websites in this book does not mean that the author or publisher endorses all of the information or recommendations of these other people's work or of their books or websites.

Contents

pages 4,5,6

Contents

Contents

Introduction

I wrote this book because I am moved and compelled by the suffering of those who have chronic debilitating Lyme and all other diseases. I live in an area that has epidemic Lyme. Almost everyone in this area knows someone who had or still has Lyme. My job as an organic vegetable farmer, an organic lawn and organic pest control for homes and landscapes service provider, has put me in an environment with opportunity to be bit by ticks with Lymes disease. A large part of the service I provide is the spraying of lawns and landscapes with organic pesticides to kill and repel ticks. Because of my exposure to Lyme ticks from my job and my love to be in the woods, I have been bit several times and have had to deal with many episodes of Lyme disease. These horrific episodes of Lyme have turned into a journey of discovery that has resulted in awesome blessings of health. I have seen many people for many years try many different methods to get well from Lyme. I have seen them try a vast array of medical antibiotics, natural antibiotics, herbs, vitamin therapies, protocols, and many different natural healing methods. Some have gotten better from these treatments and some have not. This book is for those who still need to get well. This book is knowledge from my own personal journey of defeating Lyme and knowledge of others who were Lyme sufferers and have defeated Lyme. The thought that the immune system should kill Lyme would not go away and this thought lead me to a blessed journey of learning that has brought me and others to a higher state of health. Now if I get bit by a Lyme tick it is mute no factor. Not only has Lyme been defeated but I have received a body that is more healthy, vibrant, comfortable and at peace. May this book hasten your journey to being well and at peace.

Chapter 1
Immune System Destroyers

Before we get into what things we can do to strengthen the immune system, it is important to look at the things which can reduce the function of the immune system. It is my experience that there are common things that people eat who have Lyme and other diseases that interfere with being made well. We will look at these immune destroyers and see how we can eliminate them from our life. Some of the things that I will mention may seem impossible for you to eliminate but read on because I give what I call life secrets that work to make it easier to abstain from these immune system destroyers.

Here is the list of things you should give up to strengthen the immune system.

Elimination List.

1. Eliminate sugar in all its forms. At least for a period of time while you defeat Lyme and then learn how to still eat a little sugar but keep it low and under control. It is easier than you may think. In chapter two Why Eliminate Sugar I explain how.

2. Eliminate soy, all soy products and anything with soy added, except for natto which is a fermented soybean food with the highest amount of Vitamin K2 and a super probiotic and one only needs to eat a heaping tablespoon of natto about five days a week. Some would argue other fermented soy products like miso, soy sauce, tofu and tempeh are health foods, and in small amounts maybe so, but because of their high phytoestrogens and goitrogens which can weaken the immune system they

should be avoided, especially when confronted with Lymes disease or other chronic diseases. Miso can be found made from chickpeas or sometimes called garbanzo beans and miso has a long history as a superfood. Some people may be able to eat fermented soy, but while you defeat Lyme it is best to eliminate all soy. Natto can also be made with chickpeas or black beans instead of soybeans in the Instant Pot on the yogurt setting.

3. Eliminate the gluten products: wheat, spelt, kamut, einkorn, farro, barley, triticale and rye. Even if you have been tested for gluten and the test said you can eat gluten that is not the whole story on gluten and the explanation is in the gluten chapter.

4. Eliminate corn and corn products. Some people may be able to eat some

organic corn, but while you defeat Lyme it is best to eliminate all corn.

5. Eliminate any animals fed grain and soybean. Eat 100% grass fed beef, bison, goat, and lamb. Eliminate corn, wheat, spelt, barley, and soybean fed chicken, ducks and turkey. Look for pasture raised chicken, ducks and turkey that eat insects, worms, and grass and are fed sunflower seeds, hemp seeds, oats, and scraps of beef, bison, goat, lamb and fish scraps, cheese, and yogurt.

6. Eliminate all dairy that has been fed corn, wheat, spelt, barley, rye, triticale or soybeans. A2 dairy that is 100% grass fed is good. Some people may need to avoid any kind of dairy for a short time. Read on for why in dairy chapter.

7. Eliminate anything that is not organic.

8. Eliminate anything that has artificial ingredients.

Chapter 2

Why eliminate sugar

Most people want to know what they can eat or supplement or herb they can consume to get rid of Lyme, and I have discovered that we can eat good foods, take supplements, exercise, and stay relaxed, manage stress but if we do not eliminate the bad stuff chronic Lyme or other disease may not be defeated. Fifty percent of the immune system is in the gut. What goes in the gut is very important. This part is the biggest challenge for most people that I have seen with chronic Lyme. There are certain substances that can greatly interfere with the best of treatments and protocols, and sugar may be number one. When I suggest to people struggling with Lyme or some other disease on abstaining from sugar some look at me like I am crazy or that is impossible. Their desire for sugar is so strong they think it is natural and needed to survive. This strong desire is engrained in us at an early age. Usually at a child's first birthday they are given birthday cake that has sugar and so the addiction starts. Then sugar is used to keep children occupied, as a babysitter, a comfort food, and children are rewarded with sugar thus strengthening the physical and psychological addiction. Year after year goes by and when the child, youth or adult is confronted with serious health challenges it can be hard for some to connect sugar as a culprit in disease. I do not want to take away your pleasure. I want to take you beyond what you think is a pleasure to vibrant, energetic and peaceful well-being of super health. But it's not impossible and I will show you the **powerful secret** of how to conquer the habit of eating too much sugar and other challenges. You will be easily able to say no to sugar and eventually not be tempted to eat sugar. I have heard people say to me things like "sugar makes me feel so good" "everybody eats sugar" "we need sugar to have energy" "how can something that tastes so good be so bad". Welcome to planet earth. Everything that feels good may not be good.

Before I tell you the **powerful secret** of how to abstain from sugar, I want to tell what sugar does to Lyme and some other diseases.

Sugar feeds Lyme.

Sugar multiplies Lyme.

Sugar feeds parasites - Lyme is a parasite.

Sugar weakens the immune system by almost 50%. Do you want half of an immune system? The Lyme does.

A healthy strong immune system is what can exterminate Lyme.

Now we could talk about how sugar is related to heart disease, arthritis, diabetes, poor vision, accelerated aging, obesity, non-alcoholic liver disease, cognitive brain decline, candida, yeast infections, bad intestinal bacteria, poor digestion, incomplete nutrient absorption, inflammation, allergies and some cancers but I will try to stay focused on how sugar affects Lyme. I have known so many people with chronic Lyme that have been treated by specialist Lyme medical doctors and specialist Lyme alternative natural doctors, but they are still challenged with Lyme disease for years, and one of the things that many of them had in common is they still all ate a lot of sugar and were never told by their health professional to stop eating sugar as part of wellness. I am not trying to take away your pleasure of eating sugar - I want you to have 24 hours a day of a body that feels well satisfied after eating a meal without sugar, and a healthy, vibrant, relaxed, peaceful, energetic, and Lyme free body.

Let's look at the types of sugar and their names and what I like to call sugar code names. Code names can be deceptive because at first glance one may not know it is sugar. Code names for sugar are what we need to look at in the ingredient list when we buy packaged food.

Kinds and common names of sugar and code names for sugar:

1. Agave Nectar
2. Barley Malt
3. Barley Syrup
4. Beet Sugar
3. Brown Rice Syrup
4. Blackstrap Molasses
5. Brown Sugar
6. Buttered Syrup

7. Cane Juice Crystals
8. Cane Sugar
9. Caramel
10. Carob, Carob Syrup
11. Castor Sugar, Bakers Sugar, Superfine Sugar
12. Coconut Sugar, Coconut Water
13. Coconut Palm Sugar, Coconut Nectar, Coconut Blossom
14. Confectioner's Sugar, Confectionary Sugar, Powdered Sugar
15. Corn Syrup, High Fructose Corn Syrup, Corn Syrup Solids
16. Dextrin
17. Dextrose
18. Diastatic Malt
19. Erythritol
20. Ethyl Maltol
21. Fructose
22. Fruit, yes fruit has a lot of sugar. Especially dried fruit because the sugars are even more concentrated. Sugar is sugar even if it is from fruit. It still weakens the immune system and fruit has been bred

and continues to be bred to be more sweet with higher sugar than it was years ago. Wild blueberries, cranberries and [bananas that are half green and half yellow] are low in sugar and fruits that are not ripe are low in sugar too.

23. Date Sugar
24. Demerara Sugar, Turbinado Sugar
25. Evaporated Cane Juice
26. Florida Crystals
27. Fructose
28. Fruit Juice
29. Glucose
29. Golden Sugar
30. Golden Syrup
31. Grape Sugar
32. Honey
33. Icing Sugar
34. Inulin. Research says it is a good sugar saccharide that promotes healthy gut bacteria, but with some people gut bacteria maybe unfavorably.
35. Invert Sugar
36. Isomalt

36. Isomaltitol
36. Isomaltose
36. Malt Syrup
37. Maltodextrin
38. Maple Sugar, Maple Syrup
39. Molasses, Black Strap Molasses
40. Moscovado Sugar
41. Panela Sugar
42. Raw Sugar
43. Refiner's Sugar
44. Rice Syrup
45. Sorghum Syrup
46. Sucanat
47. Sucrose, Table Sugar, White Sugar
48. Treacle Sugar
49. Yellow Sugar
50. Xylitol

Okay, how to eliminate sugar from the diet with joy!!! First we need to know why we love sugar so much. We were not born with this craving for sugar. It is not recommended to give babies under one year any sugar. I have watched many babies at their one year birthday party. They have never had sugar up until this day and I have noticed that these soon to be one year old children are usually what people would call good eaters, enjoying eating meats, dairy, grains, and vegetables. Then on their first birthday they get some birthday cake loaded with sugar, I call sugar crack because of how addictive it can be. I have seen perfectly mellow, happy, healthy babies who were good eaters. Previously they ate meat, dairy, grains and vegetables with joy and then when given sugar they turned into grumpy, fussy eaters. On their first birthday when they get a taste of birthday cake/crack they look like a cross between a starving alligator and a crazed orangutan stuffing cake and icing with both hands at light speed into their mouth with cheeks puffed out and icing in their hair, stuck in ears, dripping down the chin to their bib all the while surrounded by other sugar addicts laughing at the spectacle they only know too well. Things are never the same. AND I want to make a note here that no one has EVER died or become sick from not eating sugar. I have seen major personality changes by adding sugar to these one year old childrens diet. These one year olds that were generally content and happy most of the time, turned into children that became fussy and irritable. These children now craved sugar and soon learned that if they did not eat their meal of healthy foods meat, dairy, grains and vegetables that someone would give them something with sugar like a cookie, cake, candy, fruit juice or a sugary fruit to temporally satisfy their new addiction to keep them quiet. Another scenario is as children get older that sugar / dessert is used as a bribe to get children to eat their meal or do a chore. This so called reward of sugar reinforces that sugar is something good, going deep into the subconscious and reinforcing the addiction in the mind and body connection making the addiction even stronger. Then as the child grows, celebrations, feasts, and gatherings have sugar desserts, candy and sodas as one of the central themes reinforcing the addiction by association with a festive fun social event. Groomed to lust sugar from such a young age can make it difficult and seem impossible that one could do without sugar. Sugar also feeds and multiplies bad yeast and bad bacteria in the gut. These yeast and bacteria can locate in many different parts of the body. These yeast and bacteria signal the body they want sugar thus creating a craving for sugar in the body. People unknowingly think they have a need for sugar but it is really they have been taken captive by hungry yeast and bacteria that lust for sugar mixed with subconscious pleasure responses from an early age. The best way to bring yeast and bacteria back in healthy balance because of the overconsumption of sugar is to starve the yeast and bacteria by not eating sugar!!! YOU CAN DO IT!!! There are drugs and herbs that try and exterminate overgrowth of sugar lusting yeast and sugar lusting bacteria but they pale in effectiveness compared to starving these sugar lusting bacteria and sugar lusting yeasts by not eating sugar. When we stop eating sugar we create a whole other biosphere in the gut that is healthy and proactive. Our physiology changes from one that has been dependent on sugar to one that is not dependent on sugar. What I have seen with people who take drugs or herbs to exterminate overgrowth of sugar lusting yeast and sugar lusting bacteria is they never win the battle because they keep feeding the overgrowth of yeast and bacteria with sugar hoping that just by taking these drugs and herbs they can still eat sugar. They never get the satisfied feeling of a body without sugar. Another bad note for sugar is that when the body has too much sugar, that sugar can combine with proteins and make ADVANCED GLYCATION ENDPRODUCTS which is long for AGEs and that is what they do in the body. They create free radicals that age the body.

SECRETS ON ELIMINATING SUGAR.

NOW HERE IS ONE OF THE BIG SECRETS TO CONQUER SUGAR ADDICTION – Eat balanced meals of a protein, complex carbohydrates and good fats/oils. Yes, with the right amount of proteins, complex carbohydrates fats in a balanced healthy meal you will feel so content and satisfied it will be easier to resist eating sugar. Now at first when you quit sugar there will be a challenge to resist eating sugar because in your gut / belly are yeast and bacteria sugar lusting organisms that will put up a fuss because you are not feeding them, and your body has been accustomed to having something with sugar maybe every day for a large part of your life. But if you starve these sugar lusting yeast and bacteria they will die of starvation! Yea! Yahoo! But you must be determined to quit sugar and [you can get that determination] and with the right amount and types of healthy fats, proteins and complex carbohydrates in your well balanced meal it will be much easier, and when you starve the overgrowth of yeast and bacteria, the flora in the body will come into balance and be healthy flora, and your healthy flora will desire healthy foods and not sugar and your body will desire good food. The type of fats are very important, and don't worry fat does not make us fat, sugar makes people fat. Good fat will help the body maintain a healthy weight. Sugar is responsible for making people overweight. Now the fats must be good fat. Not ever fat is healthy fat. The good fats are 100% grass fed raw or pasteurized butter from A2 cows, 100% grass fed ghee, olive oil, coconut oil, avocado oil and red palm oil all organic of course. There is a difference between raw butter and pasteurized butter and they both have their place. When milk is pasteurized for yogurt or cheese it unlocks nutrients not available in raw milk, but raw milk has needed nutrients that cannot be found in pasteurized milk, both are vital for good health. When dairy is pasteurized many nutrients are destroyed. When I was a little kid my grandfather worked on a farm that had vegetables, fruit trees, beef, chickens, sheep and Guernsey dairy cows and so we were able to get raw milk. I did not know it at the time how good raw milk was for teeth. I never had a cavity in my teeth all through grammar school and into high school until senior year. It was not until we stopped getting the raw milk because the farm sold the dairy cows that I got one small cavity. When I had children of my own I lived in a state where we could get raw milk so my first son had raw milk and his teeth did not have any cavities and were perfect. At that time I still did not know about the benefits of raw milk for teeth. We then moved to another state that did not allow the sale of raw milk. I had another son but we only had access to pasteurized milk and then my youngest son who did not get raw milk but only pasteurized milk got cavities in his teeth. At this same time not having raw dairy I also was getting cavitation in a molar before I knew what raw dairy could do. When I went to the dentist to have my teeth checked, I told my dentist that I did not want a filling but that I was trying different nutritional strategies to fill in the cavitation. My dentist said it would never happen. But my dental hygienist who cleaned my teeth is a possibility thinker and would take pictures of my teeth every six months or so and we would look to see if the tooth was filling in or not by comparing past photos of my teeth. This went on for several years and I would try different nutritional strategies and the cavitation in my tooth was showing no sign of growing new tooth. My dentist assumed I was crazy and would just chuckle when he looked at my teeth because it still showed cavitation. But I would say there has got to be a way to regenerate teeth and I was determined to find a nutritional way to grow new tooth so my dental hygienist continued to take photos of my teeth. Then I discovered The Weston A Price Foundation and a book by Dr. Weston Price "Nutrition and Physical Degeneration".

Dr. Weston Price was a dentist that traveled the world examining indigenous peoples teeth and their diets. What Dr. Weston Price discovered was that people who drank raw milk, ate raw cheese, and raw butter had the best developed mouths and teeth with hardly ever a cavity and these same people did not have access to a dentist or practice modern dental hygiene. I then started drinking raw milk, eating raw cheese and raw butter. Then one day at the dentist's office my dental hygienist and I compared some old pictures from a tooth that had cavitation and we could see that it was filling in with new tooth. We called the dentist in to look at the pictures and he admitted that the cavitation was being filled in with new tooth and he looked at me and said what are you doing. What I was doing different was drinking raw milk, eating raw cheese and raw butter from 100% grass fed A2 Jersey cows! Now I also had been doing at that time most of what I have written in this book so I cannot say it was all the raw dairy, but for me the addition of raw dairy was the missing link to repair my teeth. If you cannot get raw dairy in your state you can buy it online and have it shipped. If your state does not allow raw dairy, it may come with a label that says not for human consumption. Even if your state does not allow raw dairy you may have the option in your state to become a member of a farm in your state that sells raw dairy which will then allow you to legally purchase raw dairy. Some farms deliver into states that do not sell raw milk because their customers have become members of the farm. To find raw butter and milk go onto realmilk.com and try raw dairy from different farms to see which ones you like the best. Benefits of butter are: Stronger immune system, more muscle strength, more endurance, nicer skin, hair, nails, stronger bones, and stronger teeth. Milk, cheese and butter from grass fed cows, goats and sheep have Vitamin K2 with butter having the highest concentration of Vitamin K2. Vitamin K2 is the truck driver for calcium and Vitamin K2 brings calcium to where it belongs like in teeth and bones and helps keep it out of soft tissue like arteries and helps prevent bone spurs. When cows eat rapidly growing green grass such as in spring and fall their butter is the most nutritious with the highest amounts of Vitamin K2. I now stock up on raw butter in the fall when the grass is green and growing fast and put it in the freezer so I can have this rich Vitamin K2 butter through the winter when the grass is not growing. Raw butter must be kept in the refrigerator because it does not keep as long as pasteurized butter. The farm I get my raw butter from recommends keeping raw butter only two weeks but I keep mine for one month then I feed it to the chickens. What about cholesterol with eating butter? I am glad you asked, and for now I will just say the latest research shows that people with high cholesterol live longer than those with low cholesterol, but that is not the whole cholesterol story and it is explained more in the cholesterol chapter. Also good fats can be ruined and cause inflammation in the body if the fats are brought to the smoke point, burned, browned or blackened because this creates free radicals that are harmful for the body. A tip for not burning/smoking oils or fats is to when frying start out with low heat and put a little bit of water into the pan with oil or fat. When the water starts to boil lower the heat to simmer, cover the pan with the lid and the steam will encapsulate the oil to keep it from burning/smoking.

Next up for healthy oils that satisfy our hunger so we do not crave sugar is olive oil. There is a lot of research on heart healthy olive oil so I will tell you what you may not know about olive oil. Buy a good brand. Many olive oils are cut with canola oil, thus turning it into something that should not be eaten. There is online research on brands that have been tested that have been cut with other oils and one's that have passed the purity test. The best olive oil in my opinion comes from Israel and Palestine. The native olive trees of Israel and Palestine are thousands of years old and the olive oil has a much richer taste than olive oil from the modern bred olive trees. Almost every meal that I have gets about a tablespoon of olive oil. Olive oil satisfies hunger for hours and nourishes and detoxifies the body. Not just fats satisfy the body but a balance of proteins, carbohydrates, and fats all together in the same meal. Sometimes if only protein and carbohydrates are eaten they may not satisfy hunger and then a desire for sugar may arise. The addition of a good amount of fat will help greatly to curb the desire for sugar. My personal favorite is olive oil and butter, but I do mix it up by having red palm oil and avocado oil too. I do not use coconut oil in my food it just does not work well inside my body, but coconut oil is a healthy oil and millions of people benefit from eating coconut oil, plus coconut oil has been found to break up Lyme biofilms in the body. I do use coconut oil on my skin. Before I shower I apply coconut oil. Then I wipe off excess with paper towels and jump in the shower. I do not wash my body with soap except for my hair. Soap dries out the skin and destroys beneficial bacteria on the skin that are part of the immune system. In my opinion, coconut oil cleans the skin better than soap, plus it moisturizes and feeds the skin nutrients.

In order to stop these sugar cravings we must eat a balanced meal every time we eat. Each meal should contain a protein like beef, bison, chicken, lamb, goat, fish or dairy. Each meal should contain a complex carbohydrate like white rice, buckwheat, oats, quinoa, amaranth, black beans, navy beans, great northern beans, red kidney beans, pinto beans, chick peas, lentils, split peas or your favorite bean. Many cultures have grains and beans together. Grains and beans together with a meal make for a more nutritious amino acid balance. Too much arginine to lysine in the body promotes the growth of certain viruses which can weaken the immune system. Grains, vegetables, fruits and many beans [not all beans] have a high arginine to lysine ration, but when we include meat, fish or dairy protein it brings the lysine up to where there is more lysine in the diet than arginine. That is one of the reasons a vegan diet is not good for long term because it weakens the immune system with a high arginine to lysine ratio. A vegan diet for about three weeks can be very good to do as a cleanse but a permanent vegan diet I do not recommended. Plus a vegan diet lacks the high concentrations of vitamins, minerals, proteins, amino acids and fats that are found in meats, fish and dairy. The beans that are high in lysine to lower in arginine are: black turtle beans, kidney beans, navy beans, pinto beans and great northern beans.

Now you have decided to give it a try and stop sugar and here are some valuable tips to help in this goal. Our words have power! When you stop eating sugar and feel those cravings rise up, do not give them more power and say "I am craving something with sugar. Or quitting sugar is hard" The body / mind will hear those words and will want to obey your words and start craving sugar more. So guard your tongue and keep your words positive. Tell your cravings to shut up, that you are in charge and those cravings are on their way out. There is great power in our words. There is quantum theory that suggests that our words and thoughts go into the quantum field and bring us back answers, strategies and concepts for what our thoughts and words desire. Also known as the Law of Attraction. This can also be looked at as all of our words and thoughts are prayers.

It's either you or [the sugar and the Lyme.] Only one wins. Show Lyme who's the boss. The other major thing to help you in your struggle to remove sugar or junk from the diet, is to not give anyone else something with sugar or any other junk food, because what we sow is what we reap. After you quit sugar do not show up to your next dinner party with a carrot cake but instead bring a bowl of steamed carrots. If we feed our family and friend's sugar addiction or other food addictions, our addictions will be harder or impossible to break. Karma catches up to everybody. But when we feed others good food, that comes back to us with good blessings and makes it much easier to accomplish our goals of quitting sugar and or other unhealthy junk food. What we sow is what we reap.

The United States has the highest consumption of sugar per person in the world and the United States has between 23,000 and 29,000 cases of Lyme reported each year. And stay away from all sugar substitutes they are poison too!

Chapter 3
Eliminate Soy

Soybeans are loaded with phytoestrogens. These phytoestrogens act as female hormones in the body throwing off the body's natural hormone balance and weakening the immune system. Soy also contains goitrogens. Goitrogens are substances that interfere with the thyroid and iodine in the body and iodine may be the most important mineral when it comes to defeating Lyme, read the iodine chapter in this book. Goitrogens are also in the raw cruciferous vegetables which are raw kale, raw broccoli, [raw broccoli sprouts do not have goitrogens], raw collards, raw cabbage, raw sauerkraut, raw mustard greens, raw radish, raw turnips, raw brussel sprouts, and raw cauliflower. When these cruciferous vegetables are cooked the lose most of their goitrogens and become superfoods. If you enjoy the taste plain, without added seasonings and oils and eat a small amount of these cruciferous vegetables raw it may be okay for you, but I see many people putting raw kale and other raw cruciferous vegetables in fruit smoothies to disguise the taste of raw kale thinking they are doing something good or dipping cruciferous vegetables into chip dip to make them taste better. But there is a reason raw kale and other cruciferous vegetable do not taste good plain. It is because our taste buds are alerting us to high goitrogens in the cruciferous vegetables. We need to cook these cruciferous vegetables which lowers the goitrogens and then brings out the superfood nutrition in these vegetables. Have you ever noticed how broccoli tastes better after a light steaming, well that is because goitrogens have been mostly removed. Some other foods with goitrogens are raw spinach, strawberries, peaches, millet, and cassava root. Cooking removes goitrogens from spinach but does not remove the goitrogens in millet. Back to soy. To make matters worse in the United States about 90% of the soybeans are GMO and heavily sprayed with the herbicide round up / glyphosate and have been coated with neonicotinoid insecticide which also kills bees and other beneficial insects. That does not mean organic soybeans are healthy, as not only does soy unbalance hormones, and the thyroid [soy is very goitrogenic,] and weakens the immune system but it is also linked to cancer. Some will argue that fermented soy is good, but the research shows that though goitrogens are reduced from fermentation there are still a lot of phytoestrogens in soy that I would not recommend eating any soy for someone who has Lyme or a compromised immune system. My one soy food exception is Natto. Natto has the highest amount of Vitamin K2 than any other food source and is super probiotic. Natto is more probiotic than any probiotic supplement I have ever taken. In Japan, children are encouraged to eat their natto like Americans encourage their children to eat their kale and spinach. One only needs to eat a tablespoon or so of this Natto superfood a few times a week to reap it's benefits. Natto helps strengthens bones and helps decalcify soft tissue. Natto also improves digestion and elimination. What's not to like about Natto? Some people do not like the taste, but to me it tastes earthy and nutritious. Give it a try. My favorite is New York Natto Organic. Natto can also be made with chick peas or black turtle beans in the Instant Pot on the Yogurt setting. There is research from Japan that consumption of seaweed which is high in iodine can negate the effects of goitrogens in Japanese fermented soy. I have not found any research for seaweed negating the phytoestrogens in soy. If you enjoy other fermented Japanese soy products eat them with discretion. The Japanese people as a race are the longest lived people. Maybe fermented soy is okay. Or okay if you are Japanese because the culture has been eating fermented soy for so long, but I would stay away from all soy while you get well from Lyme. Definitely stay away from non- fermented soy products as they are trouble for the body.

Soy is used as a cheap filler in many packaged foods and protein drinks. Miso another Japanese food made from soy that has a lot of good research behind it as a superfood also comes made with chick peas instead of soy and the chick pea miso is what I use. Another bad note on soy. A baby fed soy based formula is getting the equivalent of five birth control pills of estrogen each day. Okay Mom better breast feed your baby.

Chapter 4
Eliminate Gluten

Many people do not think they are affected
by gluten. Most likely if a person does not
have stomach bloating, constipation or
some other intestinal reaction when eating
gluten they think gluten is good for them or
okay to eat. For many years going to health
food stores and meeting all kinds of people
at health food stores and sharing health
ideas with people there were some people
that said they needed to avoid wheat. At
that time I personally thought that these
people who said they needed to avoid
wheat / gluten had the problem of eating so
much sugar that there internal bio / gut was
so out of balance that they could not digest
wheat / gluten properly and thus reacted
poorly to wheat. Fast forward many years I
had a blood allergy test and the results of
the test said I could eat wheat. I ate so
many different grains at that time that I
only ate wheat occasionally. When I saw the
allergy test said that I was good to go for

wheat I then started to incorporate more wheat bread into my diet baking my own organic wheat bread and mostly making sour dough organic whole wheat bread. Organic whole wheat bread became a staple for me as wheat became the grain I then ate the most. Then soon after my increase in wheat bread, every once in a while my stomach would bloat halfway through a meal and I could not finish the meal. I just figured it was time to fast and clean out the body. I would then go on a seven day liquids only fast. When I got off the fast my digestion seemed fine and my stomach would not bloat from eating. I would go a few years until this stomach bloating would happen again, so I would then just go on another fast with the same results of getting a digestion system that worked again. Then one year the stomach bloating came again and I decided to do a two week fast. I had always wanted to do a two week fast because research shows that the body is greatly rejuvenated at the two week mark and beyond. During a fast, enzymes for digestion leave the gut and go into the body getting rid of damaged cells that do not work or divide properly, breaking down scar tissue, releasing toxins and gunk and junk. We then get rejuvenation of the body, a rejuvenated immune system, rejuvenated hormones, cleaner arteries, cognitive function is more clear and the best stems cells on the planet made specifically for us. After my first two week fast all was well and I went on for a few more years until my stomach bloated again. I fasted again for two weeks but this time after I broke the fast, sometime during the first few days of returning to eating, my stomach started to bloat again and my stomach was not able to digest food very well. I had broken the fast with eggs and was fine eating just eggs but a few days later I started eating some kamut which is a wheat that has gluten and that is when my stomach started to bloat. I knew that I should not continue with the fast because I was too weak from fasting and from experience with fasting I know when it is time to break the fast and if I continued with the fast it would be counterproductive. I went on the internet and was looking for something that would help me with my gut that was not digesting food. I looked at an irritable bowel website that gave some ideas that may work for irritable bowel. One of the first things that was recommended was quinoa, so I cooked some quinoa, ate it and my stomach digested the quinoa just fine. Another recommendation was barley so I cooked some barley, ate it and my stomach bloated so as not to be able to finish the meal. Barley has gluten. I thought the stomach bloating problem may be gluten so I started then eating only grains that did not contain gluten like oats, white rice, quinoa, buckwheat and amaranth and I was able to eat these grains just fine without any stomach bloating or other problems. I thought oh well I guess I am now one of those people that cannot eat gluten, but I was very much thankful that I could eat again. It was a big relief to be able to eat again, especially in my weakened condition of coming off a two week fast. Interest for why I cannot eat gluten drove me to research more about gluten. I thought that only certain people had this gut problem with gluten. I looked into gluten research and found that gluten can bypass causing any discomfort in the gut but have negative effects on other parts of the body like the cardio vascular system causing enlarged heart, effecting the joints causing arthritis, causing brain fog and poor cognition. I suspect gluten can also stick to the colon for many years. I once did a cleanse that consisted of cleansing herbal tablets and a psyllium husk formula. This was before I knew anything about gluten. The instructions said to drink carrot juice along with taking the cleansing herbs and psyllium husks to see how the cleanse would clean the intestines. The cleanse instructions said the carrot juice would dye the fresh bowel movement orange except for putrid old food stuck on the intestines. I would look in the toilet after every bowel movement and I would see in many bowel movements brown and black chunks in my bowel movement along with the orange dyed fresh bowel movement. I read about an ancient wheat called einkorn that supposedly some people whose stomachs bloat when eating wheat could eat einkorn wheat. The stickiness of gluten stood out to me while making an einkorn wheat bread compared to the other non-gluten grain breads I was now making. I noticed the wheat dough stuck to the bowl, the mixing spoon and everything else. I saw clearly how very sticky are wheat dough breads. I had a home gluten test and I tested the einkorn dough for the gluten protein and the test read high for the gliadin gluten protein in wheat that causes trouble in the gut. I cannot be 100% sure, but I presume that those black and brown chunks in my bowel movement mixed with the carrot juice dyed bowel movement may have been chunks of gluten. Whatever it was I was glad to get them out. Gluten is the latin name for GLUE! Wheat paste in antiquity was used to make book bindings, papier mache and some crafts, Yikes! Many people say gluten does not bother them, but I have read research that everyone's immune system looks at gluten as an invader. Some people say spelt and some ancient wheat breads are safe to eat for people who are bothered by gluten, but I would recommend testing the dough with a home gluten test. Gluten can interfere with the thyroid uptake of iodine, and iodine could be the most important mineral when dealing with Lyme. Gluten is the latin word for glue and that is just what it does in the body sticking and gumming up. Everyone has genetic strengths and weaknesses. The evils of gluten will show up first in the weakest system of the body most times unbeknown to the person. If you are battling Lyme or some other chronic disease it is worth taking gluten out of your diet for six months to a year and see how you fair. No worries nobody ever died from not eating gluten. To give a personal example of improvement, when I stopped eating gluten is in my blood test results. I usually get yearly blood tests to see how I am doing. Before I stopped eating gluten my DHEA was low and a doctor recommended I supplement with DHEA. DHEA is a precursor in the body that makes hormones and testosterone is one on those hormones. I took DHEA for years but then started feeling bad on days I would take DHEA so I stopped. Years later when I stopped eating gluten and then had my next blood test, it showed that my DHEA was in the higher end of the Reference Interval. Years later at 65 years young, my most recent blood test shows my DHEA is higher than the Reference Interval and this is without DHEA supplementation, and my total testosterone is higher than the Reference Interval for healthy males between nineteen and thirty nine years old, which is also without any testosterone supplementation. I know that since quitting gluten my gut has healed and I can digest food much better and assume I am absorbing nutrients better too, which translates to getting more nutrition from my food. I also noticed an improvement in my thyroid after quitting gluten, and then after adding iodine to my diet my thyroid improved even more.

Chapter 5
Eliminate Corn

The first trouble with corn is that the modern hybridized corn and GMO corn have been bred to produce tons and bushels of corn for the farmer to sell and not quality nutrient rich corn for the people to eat. Research shows that heirloom open pollinated corn can have ten times the minerals as hybridized and GMO corn. Research also shows that hybridized and GMO corn does not absorb from the soil necessary minerals that humans need for health, but heirloom open pollinated corn is able to absorb these necessary for health minerals. Even if you can find heirloom open pollinated corn it has probably been contaminated with GMO corn. Corn pollen flies through the air and GMO corn pollen then breeds with other varieties of corn. Testing of organic corn in the United States shows ten to twenty percent GMO DNA in the organic corn. Some corn providers claim non GMO for their corn and this may be possible if they are extremely isolated from other farms but I have discussed this matter with people in the seed industry and it is highly unlikely in the United States that there is any corn that has not been contaminated with GMO corn DNA. When the wind blows the corn pollen flows. GMO corn seed is also coated with neonicotinoid insecticides that kills bees and other beneficial insects [it's on the label that it kills bees, and neonicotinoids are also use in home landscape products for lawns, shrubs, trees and home pest control] and then the GMO corn fields get sprayed after planting with the herbicide Round Up / glyphosate. Round Up / Glyphosate also prevents some minerals from being absorbed by the corn plant. The best heirloom open pollinated corn is probably in Russia and Iran because as of the writing of this book they do not allow GMOs in their country. The isolated home gardens in Central and South America may have pure corn too. In South and Central America they do not eat dry corn until it has gone through a process call nixtamalization which is a process when corn is boiled with calcium, lime or wood ashes which makes the niacin which is in corn available for absorption in the body and probably other nutrients too. Niacin is also known as Vitamin B3. Cultures that ate a lot of corn that did not undergo nixtamalization had high rates of pellagra which is a deficiency of niacin. Nixtamalization probably does more than just make niacin available but that is what the current scientific research shows.

I have a chicken flock that I feed sunflower seeds, hemps seeds, oats and they have access to green grass pasture, insects and worms and the chicken house is on the ground and it has a dirt floor with eight to twelve inches of hay on the dirt floor with occasional one inch of topsoil thrown onto hay which gets turned into the hay by the chickens, which makes a clean living compost pile. One side of the A frame chicken house is easily removed to allow sun light in the chicken house. I have put organic corn in a separate feeder just to see if my chickens would eat the corn and my chickens do not eat it because they prefer the sunflower seeds, hemp seeds, oats, pasture and compost pile. I have also tried feeding nixamalization corn to the chickens but my chickens will not eat that either. I have my own chickens for eggs because I do not eat corn, wheat, barley, rye, triticale or soybeans. What the chickens eat we eat when we eat the eggs. Commercial chicken feed contains mostly corn, wheat and soybeans. Commercial chicken feed also contains a plethora of added synthetic vitamins, minerals and probiotics that on the label read like a multivitamin mineral probiotic supplement. At the writing of this book most vitamins, minerals and probiotics supplements are coming from China. I do not add vitamins, minerals or probiotics to my chicken feed of sunflower seeds, hemp seeds and oats. Corn, wheat and soybeans do not fulfill the nutrient requirements for healthy chickens even when these chickens have access to pasture so vitamins and minerals must be added to commercial chicken feed. Before I learned what I know now about corn, wheat, and soybeans, I was farming chickens for meat and eggs using organic commercial chicken feed containing corn, wheat, soybeans, fish, alfalfa, grit with the added synthetic vitamins, minerals and probiotics. The chickens for meat are fed a higher protein mix with less calcium than the chicken feed for eggs. The chicken feed for eggs has less protein, but more calcium because the chickens need extra calcium for making strong egg shells. One time I ran out of the higher calcium chicken feed for the egg laying chickens which is called layer feed but I had some lower calcium chicken feed for the meat birds which is called broiler feed so I fed the egg laying chickens the meat bird feed which has the lesser calcium. After two weeks of feeding the egg laying chickens the meat bird feed, when I went to collect the eggs, when I picked up the eggs, the egg shells would break in my hands. These egg laying chickens also had access to plenty of green grass pasture, insects and worms and in the chicken house was a deep litter of leaves on the soil. When I changed back to the higher calcium layer feed the eggs did not break when I picked them up. My current flock of chickens are fed sunflower seeds, hemp seeds, fish, occasional, clabbered milk cheese, meat scraps of beef and goat with access to green grass pasture, insects, worms and a compost pile, do not need any extra calcium to produce strong egg shells. Corn, wheat and soybeans do not meet the calcium needs of a chicken so the chicken then needs supplemental calcium to produce strong egg shells. Another benefit to feeding sunflower seeds to chickens is that sunflower seeds are very high in lecithin. Egg yolks contain lecithin and when the chickens eat sunflower seeds I suspect the yolks are higher in lecithin than chicken egg yolks fed commercial chicken feed. Lecithin emulsifies fat and that is a good thing to have going on in the arteries. What the chickens eat we eat, when we eat the chicken. Some farmers advertise soy free chicken eggs and soy free chicken meat. If you look on the bag of chicken feed that is soy free the replacement for soy are peas and flax meal not flax seeds. To make flax meal, flax seeds have been crushed to remove the flax oil for sale and the flax meal is the byproduct. Flax meal has three times more phytoestrogens than soybeans and the oil in flax meal quickly turn rancid after the seeds are crushed. When flax is fed to chickens they do not gain weight as normal, and the flax oil in the meat is not shelf stable but is rancid according to the CDC. What the chicken eats we eat when we eat the chicken. It is hard to get chicken eggs that are not fed corn, wheat and soy, but having a backyard chicken flock is probably the easiest farm animal to raise. If you do a deep litter chicken house on the soil, you never need to clean it, all you do is add fresh hay now and then to cover the manure and add half to one inch of topsoil twice a year which the chickens quickly turn under the hay. This deep litter system is the way chickens were raised on commercial farms in the United States pre 1950 and some small farms are now using this method again. The deep litter turns into a living compost pile with insects, worms, beneficial mycelium, natural vitamins, minerals and antibiotics! I do start my baby chicks on organic commercial bagged chicken feed until they are two months old, but then put them on a diet of sunflower seeds, hemp seeds, oats with occasional beef scraps and clabbered milk cheese, along with green pasture, a compost pile and of course the deep litter in the chicken house. I do know a farmer that is able to raise baby chicks without using commercial bagged feed because along with her compost pile she also grows insects to feed her baby chicks. Inexpensive chicken coops and chicken coop kits can be purchased online and shipped direct to your house and you can start your own chicken flock of corn free, gluten free, soy free chicken eggs and meat! A final note on corn is that many people have developed an allergy to corn and are unable to eat animals that have been fed corn. Dry corn is famous for having various molds that can cause problems in the body. Even if you think you are okay to eat organic corn, it is worth a try to stop eating corn to see if your health improves.

Chapter 6
What Meat Not To Eat.
What Meat To Eat.

A little story first. I have a backyard flock of ducks. Baby ducks are noted for needing additional niacin in their diet until two months old, which I did not know when I first got my baby ducks, but that is another story later in this book. I thought it might be a good idea to continue adding niacin to their daily water even after two months, though it is not recommended. Several months later when the ducks started laying eggs I was continuing to add to the duck's water the recommended niacin for young ducks under two months old, even though the ducks were now about seven months old. My ducks started laying eggs and I was eating the duck eggs from my backyard flock. I then went to an allergy health professional for a maintenance checkup and had a bio scan done to look for anything that may be out of order. When finished the specialist said everything looks good except for your niacin it is way out of whack. I then thought I was apparently getting too much niacin from the duck eggs. I then told her the duck story and the niacin water. What the duck eats we eat when we eat the duck. I stopped giving the ducks extra niacin in their water. If we eat meat from beef, bison, lamb, goats that are fed the grains corn, wheat, barley, rye, triticale or soybeans we eat those grains and beans too. It is best to eat only beef, bison, lamb, goat, that are grass fed and grass finished. Grass fed and grass finished beef and bison are common now and grass fed and grass finished lamb and goats are rare but available too. Eating wild game like deer, elk, moose, caribou is very good too unless they have easy access to farms that grow wheat, barley, rye and soybeans. Eating the best meat will help the immune system do its job. Pork the other bad meat, I do not recommend eating. The pig does not detox like other farm animals. Pig holds onto toxins and store them in their fat. Even organic pasture raised pigs are going to contain toxins, it's just the nature of the pig to hold onto toxins. Just because they are on pasture and fed organic, does not mean their fat will be free of toxins because all animals when they eat produce waste products / toxins in the process of eating, digestion and utilization of food and these toxins are removed through different detox paths in manure, urine, sweating and breathing but the pig holds onto toxins more than other farm animals and these toxins are deposited in their fat. Do we really need extra toxins in our food?

The same is for fish. It is best to eat those fish with the least amount of toxins which are wild caught fish, that have fins and scales. Research shows the other sea creatures that do not have fins and scales contain more heavy metals, and high heavy metal levels in the body of Lyme patients is common. Farmed fish are fed grains and soybeans. Farmed fish are in such crowded conditions that bromide is used to exterminate the high bacteria in some fish farms. What the farm animal eats, we eat when we eat the meat. You don't need bromides. Bromides interfere with iodine in the body and iodine is an important mineral when it comes to defeating Lyme. More on this in the Iodine chaper.

Chapter 7
Dairy

Many people have dairy allergies or they are unable to digest dairy. One of the first things that gluten does in the body is destroy the body's ability to digest dairy. Gluten does this by destroying the enzyme lactase which digests lactose. Many people when they stop eating gluten usually after about six months their gut heals enough so they can again enjoy and digest dairy. Usually the first dairy that people can eat after stopping the eating of gluten are butter, cheese and yogurt. Milk is a little harder for some do digest but as the gut heals more you may be able to have milk too. Some people's guts may require about three years to fully heal from gluten destruction but need not wait that long to eat dairy, six months should be enough. Now the other possible trouble with dairy is A1 milk. A1 milk comes from certain breeds of cows like but not limited to Holsteins, Ayrshires, and breeds that have been crossed with these cows. Holstein milk and other cows that produce A1 milk have a mutated amino acid called histimine. A2 producing cows have the amino acid proline in their milk instead of histimine. Some people do not do well with A1 milk because of histimine. They may unknowingly be allergic to A1 milk. Research from Dr. Woodfork's book The book Devil in the Milk states that drinking A1 cow's milk which has histimine could cause auto immune disease, heart disease, type 1 diabetes, autism and schizophrenia. The average person may not be affected by these diseases but if one has Lyme or a weakened immune system it is a good idea to avoid A1 milk. Some cows that are A2 are Jerseys, Guernseys, Dutch Belted, and some but not all Brown Swiss cows. Camel milk is A2 but I do not recommend camel milk. There are other breeds of cows that give A2 milk around the world but these three are the most popular in the United States with the Jersey cow being the most popular and widespread A2 milk cow in the United States. Sheep, goats, yaks and water buffalo all produce A2 milk regardless of breed. If you are going to drink milk I suggest drinking 100% grass fed raw milk as it has more immune function benefits and helps build better teeth and bones than pasteurized milk. When milk is heated during pasteurizing many nutrients are destroyed. When I was a little kid my grandfather worked on a farm so we were able to get raw milk. I did not know it at the time how good raw milk, raw cheese and raw butter are for teeth. I never had a cavity in my teeth all through grammar school and into high school until senior year. And yes at that time I ate plenty of dessert with sugar. I hope you know I am not recommending eating sugar. But I still had great teeth from drinking raw milk, but I did not know it was the raw milk at that time. It was not until we stopped getting the raw milk, because the farm sold the dairy cows that I got one small cavity. When I had children of my own I lived in a state that sold raw milk so my first son had raw milk and his teeth did not have any cavities and were perfect. At that time I still did not know about the benefits of raw milk for teeth. I then moved to another state that did not allow the sale of raw milk. I then had another son but we only had access to pasteurized milk and then my youngest son who did not get raw milk but only pasteurized got cavities in his teeth. I also was getting cavitation in my molar before I knew what raw dairy could do and I told my dentist I was trying different nutritional strategies to fill in the cavitation. My dentist said it would never happen. My dental hygienist would take pictures of my teeth every six months or so and we would look to see if the tooth was filling in or not. This went on for several years and I would try different nutritional strategies and the cavitation in my tooth was showing no sign of growing new tooth. My dentist assumed I was crazy and would just chuckle when he looked at my teeth and I would say there has got to be a way to regenerate teeth. But my dental hygienist has an attitude that anything is possible, and knew I was determined to find a nutritional way to grow new tooth so she continued to take photos of my teeth. It was not until years later that I discovered The Weston A Price Foundation and a book by Dr. Weston Price "Nutrition and Physical Degeneration" Dr. Weston Price was a dentist that traveled the world examining indigenous peoples teeth and their diets. Dr. Weston Price discovered that people who drank raw milk, ate raw cheese and raw butter had the best developed mouth structure and teeth with hardly ever a cavity and they did not have access to a dentist or practice modern dental hygiene. I then started drinking raw milk, eating raw cheese and raw butter. Then at a visit to my dentist my dental hygenist compared some old pictures from a tooth that had cavitation and we could see that it was filling in with new tooth. We called the dentist in to look at the pictures and he admitted that the cavitation was being filled in with new tooth and he looked at me and said what are you doing. What I was doing different was drinking raw milk, eating raw cheese and raw butter from 100% grass fed cows! Now I also had been doing at that time most of what I have written in this book so I cannot say it was all the raw dairy, but for me the addition of raw dairy was the missing link to repair my teeth. Raw milk, raw cheese and raw butter not only build strong teeth and bones but they also support a strong immune system. The best raw milk and raw butter comes from A2 cows eating rapidly growing green grass. I can taste the difference in milk between cows eating green grass and milk from cows only eating hay. The milk tastes much sweeter and richer when the cows are eating fresh growing green grass. Butter that comes from cows eating green grass is also darker yellow than butter from cows eating just hay. When the cow eats rapidly growing green grass there is the most Vitamin K2 in the milk and even more concentrated Vitamin K2 in the butter. Vitamin K2 brings the calcium in the body to where it belongs, like to the bones and teeth and helps keep calcification from where it does not belong like in the arteries and other soft tissue. Vitamin K2 can also help decalcify a body that has been low in Vitamin K2. Plaque on teeth is calcium building up on teeth where it does not belong. Raw milk can be found on the website realmilk.com. If your state does not allow the sale of raw milk, there are farms on realmilk.com that can ship you raw milk, raw butter and other raw dairy products. If your state does not allow sale of raw milk and when the milk or butter is shipped the milk or butter may come with a label that states not for human consumption to satisfy state law. Some farms are able to delivery raw milk and other raw dairy products to residences in states that do not allow sale of raw milk but one must become a member of the farm to satisfy state law and then there is no need to have a label not for human consumption. The best raw milk, raw butter and other raw dairy products are from animals that are 100% grass fed. Some farms supplement pasture fed cows by feeding grains like corn, wheat, barley, rye, triticale and soybean along with grass pasture but the addition of grains and beans produce a milk that is higher in omega 6 fatty acids, which can make the milk and dairy products inflammatory. 100% grass fed cow's milk is higher in omega 3 fatty acids than omega 6 fatty acids which makes the milk and dairy products anti-inflammatory. What the cow eats we eat when we drink the milk. Raw dairy benefits are reduction of allergies, healthy skin, healthy hair and healthy nails. Raw dairy is also probiotic, improves immune function, and makes stronger bones, stronger muscles and connective tissue, more endurance and physical strength, and tooth cavities can be prevented or existing tooth cavities can grow and be filled in with new tooth. A2 raw dairy does a body good! Pasteurized dairy has its place in the diet too. When dairy is pasteurized different nutrients become available that are not available in raw dairy so both raw and pasteurized dairy are needed for optimum health. Most cheeses, butter and yogurt are pasteurized. But when it comes to drinking milk from my personal experience and Dr. Weston Price's research raw milk is better than pasteurized. Raw milk only stays fresh for one week. When I have one week old milk I make clabbered milk cheese. I just put the soured milk in a wide mouth jar with a pinch of rennet and let it sit on the table out of the sun until in turns into curds and whey. The soured milk does not need the pinch of rennet to turn into clabbered milk cheese but I have found that sometimes the clabbered milk will grow mold. When I put rennet in the sour milk it makes a mold free cheese all the time. I usually give this cheese to my chickens and ducks without straining through cheese cloth. The chickens and ducks really like this cheese and this was a practice of small farms years ago in the United States and still a practice in many countries that have small family farms.

Chapter 8
Eliminate Anything
That Is Not Organic

Why eat only organic. Because we want to eliminate eating any toxic insecticides, herbicides, fungicides, synthetic fertilizers and genetically, modified organisms GMOs. Plus soils that have this garbage dumped on them destroy soil life, but organic fertilizers like manure and green manure cover crops feed and multiply good soil life and that is what makes for healthy vegetables, grains and beans and good pasture and hay for livestock. Also look at things like tooth paste, bath soap, dish soap, house hold cleaner, washing detergent. We want to reduce the load of toxic ingredients we are exposed to because toxic ingredients can put a burden on the immune system. Even the clothes we wear should be 100% organic cotton, wool, hemp or bamboo. The body not only breathes through the nose and mouth, but the body also breathes and absorbs through the skin. Clothes made of polyester, nylon, rayon, acrylic, spandex are not the best choice when trying to avoid toxins. Many clothes now have teflon added to produce wrinkle free shirts and pants, and waterproofing teflon in jackets, coats, gloves and boots. The clothing tag make not say it is treated with teflon but if your cotton pants or shirt are advertised as wrinkle free or they are not soft like cotton but stiff, then they are most likely treated with teflon. Teflon has fluoride and fluoride is dangerous for the thyroid and if the body is low in iodine, fluoride can get into the receptor sites where iodine belongs and iodine may be the most important mineral when dealing with Lyme disease. See the chapter on iodine.

Chapter 9
Nuts - The Good And The Bad

If we eat only the recommended amount of nuts each day which is what can fit in the palm of the hand, than we do not need to be concerned about nuts. Eating more nuts than what fits in the palm of the hand each day can present significant challenges for the immune system. First nuts have anti nutrients call phytates and phytates are known to bind with minerals making them unavailable for use in the body. Roasting nut destroys some phytates but not all. Soaking nuts overnight in salt water and then roasting is even better to remove phytates but some still remain. The other problem for some people with nuts is the amino acid ratio in nuts of high arginine to low lysine. The ratio of high arginine to low lysine is not favorable for the immune system. High arginine to low lysine ratio favors the feeding of viruses in the body weakening the immune system. When these viruses are fed high arginine to low lysine the viruses can produce cravings for more nuts / arginine until they are starved out by not being fed nuts. Some people take a supplement capsule of lysine every day so they do not need to be concerned with this balancing act of arginine to lysine. I am not a fan of taking supplements when it can be done by eating foods. Large amounts of nuts can also be hard to digest putting a burden on the digestion which weakens the immune system. Chocolate and is very high in arginine to low lysine too.

Chapter 10
Night Shades
Are They Good For You

What and who are night shades. The night shades that people eat are tomatoes, peppers, eggplant, potatoes, okra, tomatillos, sorrel, cayenne pepper, paprika, gooseberries, ground cherries, goji berries, ashwaganda, and pepino. It seems some people can eat night shades without any problem, but others are sensitive to the alkaloids in these plants. Night shades have been linked to join pain, arthritis, gastrointestinal problems, irritable bowel, nerve sensitization, heartburn, auto immune disease, hives, skin rash, and weakened immune system. Night shades can trigger reactions in the immune system that put the body in an extremely weakened state allowing chronic disease like Lyme to flourish. If you are suffering from Lyme disease or another chronic diseases it is worth a try to eliminate nightshades from the diet. The alkaloids from nightshades can remain in the body for a while so one may need to eliminate nightshades from the diet for six months to see results, though most people will start to feel better after one month if night shades are the problem. Be patient. Somethings just need time.

Chapter 11
The FODMAP Diet
For Better Immunity

The FODMAP diet came out of Monash University and they have an app that costs only a few dollars and is worth it. Do not bother with any other FODMAP apps that are free but spend the few dollars for the real FODMAP diet app from Monash University. I have found other FODMAP information to be contrary to the FODMAP app from Monash University the founders of the FODMAP diet. FODMAP stands for Fermentable Oligosaccharides, Disaccharides, Monosaccharides And Polyols. They are a collection of short-chain carbohydrates [sugars] that are not well absorbed in the small intestine but can be beneficial in the large intestine. FODMAP's are found naturally in many foods. When some people eat too many of these FODMAP foods they can ferment in the small intestine and cause SIBO which stands for Small Intestinal Bacteria Overgrowth which causes bloating and poor digestion. Poor digestion leads to weakened immune function. When these FODMAPs in foods make it to the large intestine they are good and feed beneficial bacteria. People sensitive to FODMAP foods in the small intestine need to find out how much of these foods and which of these foods give them bloating in the small intestine. The FODMAP app is very helpful because they list foods with high, medium, low and trace amounts of FODMAP's in foods and types of FODMAP's in those foods. The FODMAP diet recommends swapping out high FODMAP foods for low FODMAP foods for two to six weeks and then gradually introduce FODMAP foods into the diet to find out which foods and or amounts of those foods are digested well. Cooking foods in a pressure cooker reduces FODMAPs in some foods. Some FODMAP foods that are canned lose their FODMAPs by leaching into the canned water such as beans. When I cook beets in the pressure cooker, I then throw out the water I cooked the beets in and then put the beets in a jar with apple cider vinegar and water. I then let the beets sit in the refrigerator for one week before I start eating the beets and I notice the difference in digestibility because the FODMAP's have leached into the water. I eat a lot of beets, sometimes every day for a week. If I only eat beets not soaked in apple cider and water once in a while the FODMAPs do not bloat my small intestine, but if I eat them every day for a week or two without soaking them in apple cider vinegar and water then I would notice bloating in my small intestine. I noticed if I drink the water the beets are cooked in for a few days in a row I can get bloating too. The canning industry uses pressure cookers for beans and other vegetables. Many people find that they are able to eat canned beans and vegetables without any intestinal distress and it is because the canning industry cooks with pressure cookers and then the beans or vegetables after they are canned are sitting in water and the FODMAP's leach out into the water while they are in the can. Always throw away the water in canned FODMAP foods if you are bothered with FODMAP's. Pressure cookers preserve nutrients and removes anti nutrients better than any other cooking method.

Chapter 12
Soup Your Next Superfood

There was a time when I was interested in the Alkaline diet. I would check my urine pH to see how different foods effected my urine pH. One of the things I learned was that when I steamed or boiled a vegetable and ate just the vegetable that my urine pH was acid. But when I drank the water that the vegetable was cooked in my urine pH was alkaline. That showed me that there are a lot of minerals in that cook water. Now when I steam, boil or pressure cook a vegetable I drink the vegetable cook water or add that mineral rich water to a soup! The vegetables that I drink the water from are low in FODMAPs because I am sensitive to some FODMAPs. I cook most of my meats, beef, bison, goat, lamb, and chicken, I cook them in a pressure cooker. Fish for me does not taste good from a pressure cooker. I cook fish on stove top or oven. After cooking meats or fish I used to throw the cook water away too, but not anymore because the same principle with cook water from vegetables applies to cook water from meats. There are a powerhouse full of nutrients in meat and fish cook water too. When we make soups with meat, fish, bones and vegetables we are getting a tremendous amount of nutrition. I like to add lentils to my soups for more nutrition. Lentils and split peas can be cooked along with the meat and vegetables. Other beans need to be cooked separately and their cook water thrown away because they contain anti-nutrients. Bone broth has become very popular. I try to have soup every day. Traditional in my family my grandmother and mother would make a meat, bone and vegetable soup and we ate that soup one day a week. The caution that I raise is that chicken feet, skin and their combs contain a lot of collagen as does beef marrow and knuckle bones. Collagen has a high arginine to lysine ratio. A balanced amount of collagen can be good, but caution should be observed when eating high collagen soups too frequently. Gelatin is made from collagen and is also high in arginine to low lysine. High arginine to low lysine ratio in the diet is known to feed viruses in the body. I was at one time eating a diet higher in arginine and lower in lysine, and I then experienced Herpes Zoster which is Shingles which comes from the Chicken Pox virus. I came to this knowledge about the high arginine to low lysine ratio from getting skin manifestations of Shingles. I had a diet high in nut butter and unbeknown to me at that time is that nuts have a ratio that is very high in arginine and low in lysine. I went to the Doctor after having what I thought were just insect bites on my head that were taking a long time to go away and I thought I should get it checked out because it might be something else. The Doctor said I had shingles and said I got there too late for treatment but she prescribed a drug anyway, but I do not remember the name of the drug but it cost $300.00 plus dollars for one bottle. I took this medicine for two days but it made me feel worse. While I was taking this medicine I got onto the internet and searched for natural cures for shingles. I came across information about how high arginine to low lysine in the diet feeds the herpes virus but high lysine to low arginine ratio prevents the virus from replicating. Since I like the nutrition approach to health, I stopped taking the drug and got some lysine and took 500mg of lysine with water before meals three times a day and stopped eating nuts and other high arginine to low lysine foods. Some recommendations for herpes virus are to take 1000mg of lysine with water before a meal three times a day when fighting a herpes virus. I made sure my diet were foods high lysine to low arginine. In three days I could feel the virus had been arrested and in three weeks the skin inflammation was gone and the nerve pain was 99.9 percent better and eventually went away not too much later. My second outbreak was when I started eating chocolate which I had not done for many years and did not know chocolate is high in arginine. I got a rash on my side and thought it maybe poison ivy or shingles. I went to the Doctor for a diagnosis and he said it was shingles. He said he would give me a prescription but I said no thanks and told him my story the last time I had shingles and had success with taking lysine and restricting arginine. He was a little defensive at first, but said that lysine does work for some people. As we continued our conversation about lysine and arginine I said that I suspected that a high lysine to lower arginine diet would suppress many more viruses and he looked at me and said he agreed. I then thought to myself that this fact is medically known but hidden for the sake of making money with drugs and other medical therapies. The older Merck Pharmaceutical Manuals have a lot of information on vitamins, minerals and other supplements and disease. Now this time instead of taking lysine I wanted to see if the rash would go away by diet along. I stopped eating chocolate and my diet is otherwise high in lysine ratio to low in arginine because I usually eat dairy, meat or fish three times a day. I also eat beans that are high lysine to lower arginine like black turtle bean, red kidney beans, navy beans and great northern beans. The rash went away. The third time I had a herpes virus manifestation was from eating a high collagen chicken broth. I usually make chicken broth starting with three quarts of water to one chicken. I wanted to make the collagen concentrated so I only put in one pint of water to a whole chicken in the pressure cooker and this chicken had the feet attached and chicken feet are very high in collagen. The chickens I buy for meat are feed a diet high in insects and pasture. The farmer I buy meat chickens from raises insects to feed her chickens and I have noticed these chickens have much more collagen than a grain and pasture fed chicken. I knew that collagen is high in arginine to low lysine but wanted to see if it would manifest herpes virus in me. After about a week or so of having this concentrated high collagen chicken broth every day, I started to develop a skin manifestation of the herpes virus. I immediately stopped eating the high collagen chicken broth and the herpes virus symptoms went away. I believe that more lysine in the diet to arginine is important for the suppression of viruses and for a more robust immune system. Before I knew this information about viruses and higher lysine to lower arginine ratio, my mother suffered from shingles for about 13 years before she died. She was taking the prescriptions and therapies of doctors for shingles for about 13 years and if I had only know then what I know now she could have been well on the road to recovery in 13 days. Higher lysine to lower arginine is not the only factor to suppress viruses, because just taking lysine has not worked for everyone because there is much more to nutrition than one nutrient. No one nutrient is Lord of all, but I believe and research shows, higher lysine to lower arginine is a crucial part of health. The meat and vegetable soups that I make are low in collagen because I like to have nutrient rich soup many times a week.

I am including here a scientific reference about high lysine to low arginine ratio and viruses. You may think you are not effected by high arginine to low lysine foods because you do not manifest any viruses, but I present this thought that the body's immune system fights to maintain homeostasis [balance] in the body but that fight eventually may be lost if we do not obey natures balance for good health. The body can and will take nutrients from itself to feed those systems in the body that are necessary for survival, but when it runs out of those stores of nutrients illness can happen. Osteoporosis is a result of the body taking minerals from the bones needed to make more immediate things function in the body like the heart beating and lungs breathing.

From my experiences with the lysine to arginine ratio I suspected that other viruses would respond the same way and that a higher lysine to lower arginine ratio in the diet is a part of the puzzle to a more robust immune system and thus better health. I searched for research to confirm my own personal findings and I came across a very interesting paper that I want to share. I was given permission by the writers of this paper to reprint their paper in this book.

Lysine Therapy for SARS-CoV-2
Christopher Kagan, Alexander Chaihorsky, Rony Tal, Bo Karlicki.
Bio- Virus Research
In this letter we report our current results using L-lysine therapeutically against SARS-CoV-2.

The first report of the clinical use of L-lysine, written by the lead author of this article, appeared in The Lancet in 1974. (1) The mechanism of action and clinical follow up confirming its effectiveness in the treatment of herpes was published in 1978 (2), and in-vitro confirmation of the inhibition of arginine by lysine was published in 1985. (3) Since then L-lysine supplementation with arginine restriction has become a recognized treatment worldwide, and the generally used dosage ranges between 100 mg to 4 grams a day; notably no toxicity has been reported with up to 8 grams per day.

(4) Lysine therapy appears to apply universally across the entire family of herpes viruses with no exceptions reported. Examples in humans include cytomegalovirus and zoster.

(2) Lysine has been shown to be suppressive in both RNA and DNA viruses, examples include the RNA-type mouse encephalomyelitis virus, and the DNA-type adenovirus type 1, SV 40, and polyoma, and the herpes virus in chickens that causes Marek's disease is known to be arginine dependent. (2) The action of lysine is complex with interference of L-arginine incorporation into the virus by L-lysine established. (2)

(3) Lysine inhibits arginine absorption in the intestine competitively lowering arginine levels, as well as inhibiting arginine reabsorption in the renal tubules. (2) A more complex mechanism with respect to SARS-CoV-2 is strongly suggested in multiple references which lay a foundation for further investigation beyond the scope of this clinical report. (6) (9) (10) (11) (12) (17) (20) (23)

A report in 2016 which included L-lysine showed a positive clinical outcome against

MERS-CoV in-vitro, although not SARS-CoV-2 which had not yet appeared. (5) Given that L-lysine appears to operate universally within the herpes viral family, it would be reasonable to expect it to work in the entire SARS viral family. Our clinical experience demonstrates effectiveness against SARS-CoV-2, and it is therefore likely to work in MERS-CoV and other members of the Coronavirus family in-vivo. Dietary lysine
2

deficiency is known to impair both antibody responses and cell-mediated immune response. (7) Lysine improves the immune system. (4)

We tested the clinical efficacy of lysine on SARS-CoV-2. Tabulated data from 40 + subjects, and non-tabulated data from 100+ subjects; 8 were in the United States, and the majority in the Dominican Republic. The age ranged between 16 to 77, with 55% of the tabulated group being female. Approximately 50% of the subjects were PCR or rapid test Covid confirmed. Approximately 50% were febrile, 30% had cough/throat, 35% anosmia, 50% CNS/muscle pain, and 45% had other symptoms.

The dose range administered was 1000 mg to 4000 mg, with the latter rarely given, and an average dose of 2000 mg. We do not recommend exceeding 3000 mg due to possible bradykinin buildup causing a cough or increasing coughing in some subjects.

(19) The dosage schedule recommended based on our study for acute cases (less than 1 month with symptoms) is a base dose of 1000 mg twice on day 1, increasing, if needed, by 500 mg to 1000 mg for a total not exceeding 3000 mg on day 2. From day 3 forward, some patients may require as high as 3500 mg. The recommended treatment times are one hour before breakfast, and 3 pm on day 1 with the times advanced earlier in the afternoon on day 2 if needed, opening a 9 pm time slot for a third dose. All doses should be taken a minimum of 1 hour before a meal, and with two cups of water. Two cups of water aids in absorption, hydration, anticoagulation, and dampens appetite which results in a decrease in the quantity of unintended arginine ingestion. A first day emergency dose of 2000 mg together (try not to exceed 4 grams in total on day 1) or a few hours apart yields outstanding results. There are many charts available of the lys/arg ratios in various foods, and a dietary ratio of 2.0 to 3.0 lysine to 1.0 arginine

for the first few days is recommended. The ratio can be lowered to 1.5 to 3.0 lysine to 1.0 arginine once near full symptom control is achieved. Restriction of coffee (and other high caffeine drinks), the importance of which cannot be stressed enough, and observing the arginine restricted diet is critical to the speed of recovery and success of treatment. Additional cautionary notes are listed at the bottom of the letter, and these cautions should be observed in follow-up clinical studies.

No trend was noted between sexes, ages, or co-morbidities in relation to lysine treatment. Approximately 80% of acute stage Covid-19 sufferers given lysine displayed a minimum 70% reduction in symptoms in the first 48 hours (not including long term symptomatic subjects). Excluding long term subjects, treatment times vary from 2 days to 3.5 weeks, with many variables at play. Patients who started lysine in the hospital were

3

discharged an average of 3 days after starting treatment. Treatment should be continued regardless of negative results, until low dose lysine is reached, and no symptoms are observed. Even when lysine was in short supply, subjects on 2 grams on day 1, and 1 gram the following days, while adhering to the dietary restrictions, had slightly delayed but timely recoveries. Resuming physical activity too early during recovery sometimes resulted in setbacks. Several of the inpatients, tabulated and non, after starting this protocol were RT-PCR negative on day 2 to 3, coinciding typically with their discharge. A larger sample size and randomized controlled trials with RT-PCR daily testing will be required to assess the true time to conversion to seronegative. Five patients who fasted on day 1, due to lack of appetite, were noted to have a significant reduction in the time and severity of febrile and non-febrile symptoms. It is assumed that zero food intake equated to no arginine consumed, and hence faster response time. For this group, the time to significant reduction in symptom varied from 4 hours to 18 hours (with only a few symptoms remaining). It is important to note that while the average subject may be completely asymptomatic on day 3 or 4, if they stop treatment/exhaust lysine supply, on many occasions, symptoms return, albeit usually reduced in severity. Typically for this group, symptoms abate within a few hours of resuming their lysine.

Lysine is a treatment, not a cure, and is dependent on the immune system response gathering momentum to further control the illness. All should remain on at least a maintenance dose of 1 gm for a minimum of a 1 week (preferably 2 weeks or more) after all symptoms have abated including following dietary restrictions for 3 weeks to prevent relapse. Evidence of asymptomatic clotting for those who stopped the regimen too early was observed. Coffee (associated arginine increase) can overwhelm lysine rendering it ineffective until the caffeine effect subsides. The caffeine effect displaces lysine from the metabolic pathways. (18) Coffee/high caffeine consumption was the most common behavior of long term symptomatic subjects, followed by a vegetarian/lysine deficient diet and exercising. Coffee/high caffeine drinks should be avoided during treatment and for 3 weeks after recovery at a minimum. Our treatment protocol has been used in more than 180 patients, with 40+ reported here. Only 1 subject was hospitalized after starting lysine for secondary bacterial infection. He was discharged 6 days later, with no long-term effects. One Covid-19 confirmed fatality due to secondary bacterial infection occurred. Obviously more studies, including randomized controlled trials, are required for full clinical understanding.

One of the most important observations in relation to lysine was the incredibly short time to eliminate/reduce fever presumably due to extinguishing the associated cytokine storm. Cytokine storm appears to be extinguished in hours, based on the 5 inpatients

4

who appeared to be in severe crisis when lysine was administered who showed very rapid reduction in symptoms and stabilization. CRP levels returned to normal, yet D-dimer levels were high in some subjects. Only a small percentage of subjects on lysine were febrile past 24 hours, and most were relieved in less than 12 hours with proper doses and dietary restrictions. IL-10 inhibits the synthesis of IL-6, TNF and IL-1 beta which are implicated in fever. (8) IL-10 serves as an endogenous antipyretic. (8) Lysine deficiency raises IL-6 inflammatory cytokine levels, so lysine potentially has an IL-6 inhibitory effect, and lysine also increases IL-10 anti-inflammatory cytokines as shown in the liver. (7) Therefore, it is logical to assume that supplementation with lysine could restore or augment IL-10 levels resulting in downregulating proinflammatory cytokines, in turn eliminating fevers and cytokine storms. IL-6 inhibitors for patients with severe Covid-19 are associated with decreased intubation, reduced mortality, and increased discharge. (13) L-lysine decreases nitric oxide production (14), thereby limiting a key role in the pathogenesis of inflammation, and thus lysine may serve an anti-inflammatory role (15) by reducing pro-inflammatory cytokines (24). These clinical results suggest that lysine appears highly suppressive of viral replication, and if these results are confirmed by further studies, lysine should significantly flatten the curve, reduce mortality and hospital bed utilization while we await a curative vaccine or vaccines, ideally one with universal application across the entire Coronavirus group.

It might be that the combination of suppressive lysine and vaccination is superior to either alone. There may be places in the world where even inexpensive lysine is unaffordable, but high lysine foods combined with arginine restriction might still serve the purpose. Our hope is that these findings will encourage those in a position to perform follow-up studies to do so, hopefully confirming its usefulness, and further refining our understanding of optimal dosage, mechanisms, routes of administration and how to maximize the efficacy of this therapy.

Cautionary note: Long term asymptomatic (over 1 month) and medically fragile patients
should exercise caution and use low dose lysine for the initial days and incrementally
raise their dose 500 mg every 4 to 5 days, until reaching 2500 mg daily and evaluate.
Higher doses have been used, but the concern is that doses higher than 3000 mg could
result in occult clots embolizing. No coffee, exercise, marijuana, or arginine rich foods
during treatment is included in the recommended protocol. Lysine has been reported to
nearly double serum zinc levels without supplementation. (16) Zinc and calcium should
not be given with lysine since lysine also raises calcium levels. (22) Patients on
pacemakers should be under close clinical observation since lysine might increase
cardiac output (21) and increases pulmonary resistance. (14) Clinicians who are
5

interested in more details may contact us for additional information at Bio-Virus
Research +1(775) 742 8811,
xyz1953@gmail.com).
Bio-Virus Research Inc.
5774 Tappan Dr.
Reno, Nevada, USA
xyz1953@gmail.com
+1(775) 742-8811

1   Kagan, C.; Lysine therapy for herpes simplex. Lancet i: 137 (1974).

2.   Griffith, R. S.; Norins, A. L.; Kagan, C.; A multicentered study of lysine therapy in herpes simplex infection. Dermatologica 156:257-267 (1978).

3.   Griffith, R. S.; DeLong, D. C.; Nelson, J. D.; Relation of arginine-lysine antagonism to herpes simplex growth in tissue culture. Chemotherapy 27: 209-213 (1981).

4.   PubChem (internet). Bethesda (MD) National Library of Medicine (US), National Center for Biotechnology Information; 2004- Pubchem compound summary for cid 5962, lysine; (cited 2020 aug. 28) available from: http://pubchem.ncbi.nlm.nih.gov/compound/lysine.

5.   Muller, C.; Kari, N.; Ziebuhr, J.; Pleschka, S.; D, l-lysine acetylsalicylate + glycine impairs coronavirus replication. Journal of Antivirals & Antiretrovirals 8(4) 142-150 (2016).

6.   Riley, F. L.; Martin. L.; Morin, E. L.; Stephens, E.E.; Hilton, B. L.; Polyriboinosinic-polyribocytidylic acid-poly-l-lysine (poly(icl) without carboxymethylcellulose (cmc): a

new primate-effective interferon inducer. Proceedings of the Society for Experimental Biology and Medicine 169: 183-188 (1982).

7.   Han, H.; Yin J.; Wang, B.; Huang, X.; Yao, J.; Zheng, J.; Fan, W.; Li, T.; Yin, Y.; Effects of dietary lysine restriction on inflammatory responses in piglets. Scientific Reports 2451 (2018).

8.   Leon, L.R.; Kozak.; W., Rudolph, K.; Kluger, M. J.; An antipyretic role for interleukin-10 in
LPS fever in mice. Am. J. Physiol. 276 (1999).

9.   Heurich, A.; Hofmann-Windkler, H.; Grier, S.; Liepold, T.; Jahn, O.; Pohlmann, S.; Tmprss2 and adam17 cleave ace2 differentially and only proteolysis by tmprss2 augments entry
driven by the severe acute respiratory syndrome coronavirus spike protein. Journal of Virology 88: 1293-1307 (2014).

10. Saito, S.; Matsui, S.; Wantanabe, M.; Waga, T.; Kajiwara, Y.; Shirota , M.; Iijima,
M.; Kitabate, K.; Matsushita Y.; Moriguchi, I.; Inhibitory activity and protein binding of L-lysine derivatives as angiotensin converting enzyme
inhibitors. Arzneimittleforschung 1078-81, 1990.

11. Melen, K.; Kinnunen, L.; Julkunen I.; Arginine/lysine-rich structural element is involved in

interferon-induced nuclear import of STATs. J. Biol. Chem. 16447-55 (2001).

6

12. Baral, R.; White, M.; Vassilliou, V. S.; Effect of renin-angiotensin-aldosterone system inhibitors in patients with covid-19; a systemic review and meta-analysis of 28,872 patients. Current Atherosclerosis Report 22, 61 (2020).
13. Sinha, P.; Mostaghim, A.; Bielick, C. G.; McLaughlin, A.; Hamer, D. H.; Wetzler, L. M.; Bhadelia, H.; Fagan, M. A.; Linas, G. P.; Assoumou, S. A.; Leong M. H.; Lin, N. H.; Cooper, E. R.; Brade, K. D.; White, L. F.; Barlam, T. F.; Sagar, M.; The Boston medical center covid-19 treatment panel.; Early administration of interleukin-6 inhibitors for patients with severe covid-19 disease is associated with decreased intubation, reduced mortality, and increased discharge. International Journal of Infectious Diseases 99: 28-33 (2020).
14. Carter, B. W.; Chicoine, L. G.; Nelin, L.D.; L-lysine decreased nitric oxide production and increases vascular resistance in lungs isolate from lipopolysaccharide-treated neonatal pigs. Pediatric Research 55: 979-987 (2004).

15. Sharma, J.N.; Al-Omran, A.; Parvathy S. S.; Role of nitric oxide in inflammatory diseases. Inflammapharmacology 15(6): 252-259 (2007).

16. Rushton, D.H.; Nutritional factors and hair loss. Clin. Exp. Dermatol. 27(5): 396-404 (2002).

17. Ismawati, R.; Wirdjatmadi, B.; Priyatna, Y.; Mertaniasih, N. M.; The effect of zinc, lysine, and vitamin A supplementation to increase cellular immune response of pulmonary tuberculosis patients. Biochemistry & Physiology: open access 55:2168 (2015).

18. Nikolic, J., Bjelakovic, G.; Stojanovic, I.; Effect of caffeine on metabolism of l-arginine in the brain. Mol. Cell. Biochem. 244:125-128 (2003).

19. Taddei, S.; Bortolotto, L.; Unraveling the pivotal role of bradykinin in ace inhibitor activity. Am. J. Cardiovasc. Drugs 16(5) 309-321 (2016).

20. Boldt, A.; Gergs, U.; Frenker, J.; Simm, A.; Silber, R-E; Klockner, U.; Neumann, J.; Intropic effects of l-lysine in the mammalian heart. Naunym Schmiedebergs Arch. Pharmacl. 38 0 (4): 293-301 (2009).

21. Li; Wenhui & Wong.; Fang & Kuhn.; Jens & Huang.; I-Chueh & Choe.; Hyeryun & Farzan, M.; Animal origins of severe acute respiratory syndrome coronavirus; insight from ace-s-

protein interactions. Journal of Virology 80: 4211-4219 (2006).

22. Civitelli, R.; Villareal, D.T.; Agnusdei, D.; Nardi, P.; Avioli, L.V.; Gennari.; C. Dietary L-lysine and calcium metabolism in humans. Nutrition 8(6): 400-405 (1992).

23. Almansour, H.; http://www.researchgate.net/publication/34033 4873coronavirus prophylaxis (the role of lysine amino acid in the prevention of viral attachment to the human cells). 4 (2020).

24. Kankuri, E.; Hamalainen, M.; Hukkanen, P.; Salmenpera,P.; Kivilaakso,E.; Vappatalo, H.; Moilanen, E.; Suppression of pro-inflammatory cytokine release by selective inhibition of inducible nitric oxide synthase in mucosal explants from patients with ulcerative colitis. Scandinavian Journal of Gastroenterology 38: 186-192 (2003).

In summary eat your soup, because we get nutrients from soup we may not get anywhere else. Soup does a body good!

Chapter 13
Exercise Made Easy

When challenged with Lyme or some other chronic disease exercise is important. Exercise can be fun and easy and should be fun and easy. Many people think that in order for exercise to do anything there must be pain or discomfort. This is far from the truth. Exercise should always be fun and easy unless you are an athlete and are training for a specific sport then you are going to hurt, but exercising like an athlete can compromise the immune system. If we exercise too hard or too much the body needs to recover from that hard exercise. The body needs to repair the damage that was done during exercise and replenish the nutrients that were used during exercise and lost during sweating. If we exercise too hard or too much the body will take energy to repair and replenish what was lost during hard exercise and sacrifice energy needed for other things in the body like the immune system. What we are looking to do is enhance the immune system with exercise. I have an exercise rule and that rule is "that exercise should always give us more energy for our day and never take away any energy for our day." The Lyme patient has a load of toxins in the body and exercise will help move those toxins out of the body. The first exercise I would recommend is rebounding. Rebounding works the lymph system by the action of jumping up and down. Jumping/rebounding is a great way to get the lymph system going and only requires two or three minutes a day. Rebounding activates the lymph system and will help remove toxins from the body. It sounds too simple but rebounding is very powerful and you only need two or three minutes a day to get that lymph system moving. When rebounding it is not necessary for your feet to go into the air and leave the rebounder to work the lymph system. Just gently bounce. If you have ever seen a one year old baby do the baby bounce that is what they are doing working the lymph system. All one needs is two or three minutes a day on a rebounder to get the benefits of stimulating the lymph system and thus by rebounding we are taking out the trash/toxins collected in the lymph system. Do not overlook rebounding because it is a most powerful exercise to help regain health and then to keep health. If you have been sedentary, rebounding is an easy way to ease into an exercise program. To show the power of rebounding I want to share a story. I had these small crusty growths on my head that would not go away. I would scrape them off my head and they would grow back. I went to the dermatologist to find out what they were and if they were dangerous. The dermatologist said it was seborrheic keratosis and it was genetic and there was nothing I could do about it. I kept having this thought that it was just toxins in my body. Soon after this I bought a rebounder because of what I had learned about rebounders and the activation of the lymph system. The first day I used the rebounder was for seven minutes and when I got off my head felt a little dizzy. The slight dizziness stayed throughout the day but did not prevent me from working or driving. The next morning I did not feel any more dizziness. It was later that week that I was searching for more information on the lymph system and saw a video that explained that just recently lymph nodes were discovered in the top of the head. I continued to rebound almost every day and after about a year all the seborrheic keratosis growth were gone and have never come back! The next type of exercise to do is light and easy cardio exercise which slightly elevates the heart beat like walking, jogging, cycling, and swimming. Light and easy cardio exercise stimulates the immune system, improves blood circulation and has been shown to lengthen telomeres. One does not need to huff and puff hard to get in a good cardio workout. Actually I recommend only bringing a cardio workout to a level where the heart rate is slightly raised but you are able to breathe through the nose comfortably with the mouth closed and your body feels comfortable, not any pain. If you need to open the mouth to get more oxygen then slow down your exercise and keep it light and easy so all you need is to breathe comfortably through the nose with the mouth closed. This way you will not over train because overtraining puts too much stress on the body and the body can only do so much and the body has to pick where it needs to send its limited energy and other body systems may be compromised like the immune system. For some people jogging or fast walking may be too much and for those people I say just go for a normal comfortable walk and you will get great benefits too! I used to jog for years and benefited greatly but now I enjoy walking much more and have found I have more energy for my other daily tasks. Each of us needs to find what works best for us. I personally usually walk for thirty minutes a day first thing in the morning. There are many studies that say walking is better than jogging but I think it really gets down to the individual and what is best for them. Get cleared by your physician before starting any exercise program and start out slow and easy for just a few minutes like three or five minutes at the most when starting a cardio exercise. Just going for a gentle walk is awesome. As you feel more comfortable raise the time doing cardio exercise to ten minutes and if you like up to twenty minutes. For jogging I think 20 minutes is the max and no need to jog for more time because I think it is then a waste of energy with no benefits for the immune system but could be counter productive. When walking no more than 30 minutes is needed for good health. If you need to bring in oxygen through the mouth you are exercising too fast and need to slow down. Another exercise rule that I mentioned before is that exercise should give you more energy for your day and never take energy away from your day. If after exercising you are tired and lack energy for your day then back off from how much you exercise. No need to go over twenty minutes of cardio to get the benefits of an improved immune system. If you can't get up to twenty minutes of cardio just do whatever is comfortable for you. Just going for a normal or comfortable brisk walk could be all the exercise you may need. There is a lot of research that says going for a 30 minute easy walk is more beneficial than jogging. Work within your own energy supply. Keep exercise easy and fun, but just do something. A word on high intensity interval training which has become popular in many circles. I know people who think they must continually train harder and harder but this is not good. There are too many things that can go wrong with high intensity interval training. High intensity interval training is running or cycling at full speed for thirty seconds and then walking or coasting for ninety seconds and doing this for a total of eight times or less. This type of training has shown gains for athletic performance but there is no research on long term health studies for longevity and I would suspect there will never be. I had an acquaintance that used to race horses and I asked her how many years do racehorses race. Racehorses run close to full speed during a race on a one mile racetrack. On a one mile race track the race can be under two minutes. She said that race horses raced for about two or three years and then they went out to pasture because she said the race horses had multiple injuries and needed care. She also had a farm that tended to these injured race horses. I had another acquaintance that had horses that gave trail rides. These horses just walked leisurely along a path through the woods. I asked her how long the horses are good for giving trail rides and she said twenty years. I then thought the turtle wins the race and that is how I should exercise. Galapagos tortoises live over 150 years and some over 200 years. Ever notice how slow they move. They take it easy. No rush. I have never seen any centurions doing high intensity interval training. I also had a relative who did high intensity training, he called them wind sprints. He had a heart attack one day after doing some high intensity training/wind sprint exercise. After a few years recovery time from the heart attack and under doctors care, he started doing high intensity training exercise/wind sprints again. One day a neighbor found him lying on the road after doing high intensity training exercise/wind sprints but they could not revive him. Keep your exercise fun and easy. Elite athletes in general do not live as long as the average person because they push their bodies so hard. The next exercise I recommend is weight lifting and body weight exercises. I personally like pushups, chin ups, crunches, squats, barbell and dumb bell exercises like curls and overhead press. I like exercises that engage the whole body. I traded my bench press for pushups and my lat machine for chin ups and never looked back. I notice how that change has benefited my spine, strength and overall health. I do not do chin ups at full arm extension because I believe that is putting too much stress on the shoulder joint. When I do pushups I do not let my shoulders arch back but keep them level or in front of my body which prevents getting too much stress on the shoulder joints.

When I do the overhead press I do not lift to full extension over my head. Maxing out the joints is popular during all kinds of workouts, but very bad ergonomics that stress the joints. I worked in construction many years as a mason lifting blocks, bricks, buckets of concrete, pushing wheel barrows of cement, climbing scaffolds and ladders. When working in construction no one maxed out the joints when working. If we did we would not last very long before there was some kind of injury. Many people exercise with full range of motion and max joint extension which I think is a mistake for many exercises. I think the bench press is bad for the spine because a lot of the weight is being supported by the ribs transferring the weight to the spine in an unnatural way. Pushups are much better because they engage the whole body structure. Dead lifts can be bad for the back, I do not recommend them it's just not worth it. I feel that just doing squats with light weight or even no weights gives the same benefits as dead lifts without the risks of injuring the back. Farm and gardening work are great exercises too! I will not go into all the pros and cons of different weight lifting exercises but correct form weight bearing exercise with moderate intensity will improve immune function. The goal here is not to build large amounts of muscle mass but to work at an intensity to stimulate health. When we do weight bearing exercise muscle mass and tone can increase but that is not the primary focus. Building a fit, healthy body with a strong immune system is the goal. Try to find a sensible fitness coach to teach you how to exercise and or get some exercise books and just start exercising with caution. Listen to your body. It has taken me many years of exercise to find out what is good and works for me and I am always open to more improvement. A key is knowing how much to exercise. Exercise should always give you more energy for the day and not rob you of energy for your day. If exercise ever robs you of energy for the rest of your day you are doing too much and it will definitely show up in a weaker immune system. Learning how much to exercise will come with experience. Next exercise is Tai Chi and Static Standing Qigong which are very powerful exercise to help release tension and relax the body. We may not know or feel how much tension we carry in our bodies and Tai Chi and Standing Static Qigong are powerful exercises to help relax the body and enhance the flow of chi. In Tai Chi and Qigong they say if you do Tai Chi and Qigong every day you lay down one piece of paper and at the end of the year you have a stack of 365 pieces of paper. What that means is that the benefits of Tai Chi and Qigong are accumulative over the years. I have been doing Tai Chi almost everyday for 20 years and can testify to that fact. The slow movements of Tai Chi allow us to feel the energy in the air and the slow relaxed Tai Chi movements allow us to tune in more with feeling chi flow in the body and releasing blockages and tension in our bodies. When doing Tai Chi think of it as swimming in air and you will feel what I am talking about. Standing Static Qigong sometimes called Standing Like A Tree is another immune booster that helps build and circulate chi in the body. Just doing 10 minutes a day of Standing Static Qigong can give many benefits. Tai Chi and Qigong may sound very esoteric but it is a science based Chinese exercise to help balance what the Chinese call Yin and Yang. Yin is soft and Yang is hard. Most people are too hard [tense] and need to soften relax more. In Tai Chi they say we are to search to for [song] in the body. [Song] in Tai Chi means open relaxation in movement, when holding a still posture and in daily life of whatever we are doing. This is Yin Yang harmony. The soft open relaxation balanced with the hard contraction is Yin Yang harmony. The more relaxed we are the better are bodies function and the better our bodies regenerate to make new cells and a stronger immune system. High level athletes know this principle well, but they call it relaxed tension. When athletes find the relaxed tension while doing their sport they perform that sport much better. Doing Tai Chi can help develop relaxation in the body, Yin Yang harmony, hard clothed with the soft, or as they say in Tai Chi, steel clothed in cotton. Being relaxation in our daily life, chores etc. is very healing to the body. As you develop a practice of Tai Chi and Qigong you will find yourself bringing the relaxed feeling from Tai Chi into your daily life. Another powerful exercise is the ancient Chinese art of Bagua circle walking. Bagua is related to Tai Chi and Qigong. Bagua consists of walking in a circle using different stationary palms. As we walk the circle with stationary palms, it is easy to feel the energy in the air and the circulation of chi in the body. Bagua can be a way to get your daily walk in while opening meridians in your body and building a store house of chi. I need to say that many Bagua books and schools describe circle walking with the upper body twisted to the inside of the circle and the feet shuffle along sliding on the floor. This is erroneous because that is bad ergonomics for the spine. Always keep the upper body square with the lower body and walk normal while holding the different palms of Bagua and you will reap the benefits. The feet shuffling on the floor walk comes from the misunderstanding of what they call in Bagua mud walking. The real meaning of mud walking is where the practitioner tries to develop a sensitivity to feel the energy in the air on the lower legs while walking the circle, like one would feel walking through mud, thus the phrase mud walking. In Tai Chi, Qigong and Bagua it is a goal to feel the energy in the air with the body. Cheng Man Ching a famous Tai Chi teacher that brought real Tai Chi to the United States would say Tai Chi is like swimming in the air. At first it is easy to feel the energy in the air with the palms of the hands. As one's Tai Chi practice continues in time that sensitivity grows from the palms to the whole hand, to the arms and other parts of the body with the goal of being able to feel the energy in the air with the whole body. Feeling the energy in the air is one of the goals in Tai Chi, Qigong and

Bagua and feeling this energy with the body increases [song] open relaxation in movement. Some Tai Chi exercises have twisting movements where the upper body twists from side to side and the lower body is stationary. This is also long term bad for the spine and best to avoid these twisting exercises. Yoga is another good exercise that can benefit the health of the body that can help open up and relax the body to enhance circulation and immune function. Just don't push the stretch too far. It is better to just relax into the posture and only go as far into the yoga posture as is relaxingly comfortable. Yoga should not be a competition on how far one can stretch. More is less and less is more. Be careful if doing hot yoga. I did Bikram hot yoga for about three years, three times a day. I really pushed myself hard during the 90 minute 105 degree heated class. Many of the Bikram Yoga postures are isometric muscle working postures while stretching at the same time and I pushed hard with all the postures. It was not uncommon for people to leave the heated room during class to cool down. I brought a half gallon of water into class and drank the whole thing during class, and the towel I was standing on during class was completely wet from my sweat when we were finished with class. After class I need to hydrate more. I felt really good after class and this became additive for me. After three years I hit a wall in class and could not take the heat in class that I so loved before. A little sweating is good, but pushing myself hard in yoga postures and profusely sweating three times a week in 105 degree heat was way overboard for me. Over sweating can deplete minerals stores from the body that can take years to replace. It took me years to recover from my escapades with hot yoga. Hot yoga can be great but in moderation.

In summing up we need exercise for good circulation and when we put a slight demand on the body it triggers health in the body. We were made for physically active lives and if we become sedentary, we use it or lose it and the immune system suffers too.

Chapter 14
The Skin Brush Detox

The skin brush detox is a powerful way to stimulate the lymph system thus helping to move toxins from Lyme and other environmental toxins out of the body. Even the process of eating the cleanest organic food and then the process of digesting and burning food as fuel in the body produces waste products that must be eliminated from the body. Skin brushing is often overlooked as a powerful healing practice, but when you give it a try you will notice how after a skin brushing session of about five minutes one feels invigorated. After about a week of daily skin brushing you will notice your skin becoming smoother, moister and dry patches disappearing and all the while moving toxins out of the body. Skin brushing helps remove the dead layer of skin allowing the skin to breathe better too. Start with skin brushing three days a week but find your own schedule on how much skin brushing is good for you. Skin brushing before a shower is good but never skin brush in the shower or after a shower with wet skin.

Chapter 15
Iodine Could Be
The Most Important Mineral
To Defeat Lyme

In the years before the 1970s in the United States, iodine was added to grain flours and those flours were used to make bread and other baked goods. Early in the 1970s iodine in flour and bread was replaced by bromide. Bromide is goitrogenic meaning it disrupts the production of thyroid hormones by interfering with iodine uptake in the thyroid gland. Bromide is toxic to the body and if the body does not have adequate stores of iodine then bromide will take its place in the body and wreak havoc. The thyroid is a place where iodine accumulates the most and if the body does not have adequate iodine then bromide will takes its place causing the thyroid to not function properly. Iodine has also been found in every cell of the body. According to reference:

https://www.ncbi.nlm.nih.gov/pmc/articles/PMC3509517/ website, in the United States data from large population studies have shown that medium urinary iodine levels decreased by approximately 50% between the early 1970s and the early 1990s. The first recorded Lyme disease cases in the United States were in the city of Lyme Connecticut in 1975. I repeat in the early 1970s iodine in flour and bread was replaced with bromide and then the first record cases of Lyme in the United States were in 1975. Is there a connection here, I think so from my own use of iodine and Lyme journey and others suffering with chronic Lyme that I have shared how iodine can help the body to defeat Lyme and they have used that information and are now taking iodine and have defeated Lyme. Adequate levels of iodine must be in the body for good immune health.

As of the writing of this book there is no generally agreed upon iodine test that can evaluate how much iodine should be supplemented. I hear many times from those suffering from Lyme "my doctor tested me for iodine and said my iodine levels are good". If there is no generally agreed upon iodine test that can evaluate iodine dosing this is a disservice to the patient. Plus iodine levels have dropped 50% between the early 1970s and 1990s so doctors are evaluating their dosing or non-dosing of iodine looking at the present average population iodine levels which were 50% less in the 1990s than pre early 1970s and now may be less in the year 2021 because there is more bromide and fluoride in the environment than was years ago that can lodge in the thyroid if there is not adequate iodine in the diet. Plus there is presently now more bromide and fluoride in foods and drinks. Healthy iodine levels cannot be judged by the current status quo. If one does not get adequate iodine then bromide and fluoride will takes iodine's place in the body with disastrous results. There are three current tests for iodine: a urine test, another is a plasma test, and the third is an iodine loading test. The iodine loading test is when a high oral dose of iodine [usually 50mg of Iodoral which is iodine and iodide] is taken and then iodine is measured in the urine to see how much comes out in a twenty four hour period. The iodine loading test presumes that depending on how much iodine the body retains or expels in the urine that an approximant iodine dosing rate can be prescribed. The iodine loading test has been able to point many people in the right direction for iodine dosing, BUT there are also a population of people that are sensitive to large amounts of iodine and or are so full of toxins and especially bromide and fluoride which compete with iodine for receptor sites in the body, that when this sensitive population takes 50mg of Idoral they may suffer rapid uncomfortable detoxification symptoms such as lethargy, headaches, and heart palpitations. The best way in my opinion to find your optimal iodine dose is with the liquid atomic nascent iodine that Edgar Cayce developed. There are three Nascent Iodine's I recommend: Enviromedica Nascent Iodine which at the time of this writing is made from seaweed but works differently in the body than just eating seaweed, Iodine Edge Nascent Iodine and Detoxadine Nascent Iodine which are made from deep earth minerals of potassium iodide but works differently in the body than just taking potassium iodide. Detoxadine Nascent Iodine has the most iodine per drop but I recommend starting out with a lower dose Nascent Iodine like Enviromedica Nascent Iodine or Iodine Edge Nascent Iodine. Idoral is a popular source of iodine and consists of iodine and potassium iodide in a 12.5mg or 50mg tablet but is not a nascent iodine product and I have no personal experience with this product but it is very popular. Another popular source of liquid iodine but is not a Nascent Iodine is Lugols solution which is iodine and potassium iodide. Lugols solution was a very popular go to medicine in doctors offices pre 1950s. Iodine was discovered in 1811 and soon thereafter entered doctors offices. Iodine was used up to about 1950 for treating dermatologic conditions, chronic lung disease, fungal infestations, syphilis, [syphilis is similar to Lyme in that syphilis and Lyme are both a spirochete] arteriosclerosis, curing goiter, as a disinfectant, and more. The Nobel laureate Dr Albert Szent Gyorgi wrote: " When I was a medical student, potassium iodine was the universal medicine. Nobody knew what it did, but it did something and did something good." In 1851 the French chemist Chatin discovered that iodine cured thyroid goiter. In 1924 the Morton Salt Company added iodine to salt at the request of the United States government because thyroid goiter was a problem in the United States. Can you just eat seaweed for iodine? Maybe but if you are severely low in iodine and have toxins stuck in the body [some toxins can only be removed by iodine] Nascent Iodine can be very helpful in allowing you to quickly PHYSICALLY FEEL your need for iodine much more easily than just eating seaweed or other iodine supplements, and if digestion is compromised iodine from seaweed or other foods may not be sufficiently absorbed, whereas Nascent Iodine is easily absorbed. Nascent iodine is made through a special electronic process that makes the iodine much more available and rapidly available in about one to three hours which makes it VERY EASY to know if you need iodine and how iodine is affecting you because it works so rapidly. Most people are able to feel the effects of nascent iodine quickly as an increase in energy within a few hours of taking nascent iodine. If you drink coffee, green tea or other caffeinated drinks it may be harder for you to feel the effects of Nascent Iodine at first because the caffeine rush is so strong and the Nascent Iodine energy is a little more subtle, but caffeine drinkers I know report back that they do notice an overall energy increase from Nascent Iodine throughout the day and some have been able to cut back or eliminate their need for caffeine. If you have cold hands and feet, or low body temperature, or mental fog, or anxiety, or constipation, or if you have Lyme, or another chronic disease, or you feel a lack of energy you should try supplementing with iodine. Even if you do not have any of those symptoms you should try Nascent Iodine just to see if your health improves. Start slow, start slow, start slow with any iodine product. Take Nascent Iodine or any iodine supplement only first thing upon arising in the morning because Nascent Iodine may give you too much energy to go to sleep if taken later in the day. Put one drop in a glass of water and drink only one quarter of the glass of water [that is taking a quarter drop of Nascent Iodine]. See how you feel. It may take two or three days of taking Nascent Iodine to feel anything, which would be a boost in energy or warmth over the body with diminishing disappearing cold hands and feet, normalized body temperature, clearing of mental fog and reduction or elimination of anxiety or other Lyme symptoms. If you do not feel anything drinking a quarter drop of iodine a day than the following week increase your dose to a half drop a day and if you still do not feel anything the next following week increase to one drop a day. If you still do not feel anything, up the number of iodine drops by adding one drop a day each week until you feel something good up to only the recommended amount of drops as listed on the bottle of Nascent Iodine. I recommend this slow approach taking iodine because everyone is different in how they need and utilized iodine, how deficient in iodine they may be, and how toxic they may be with bromide, fluoride, Lyme, heavy metals, other toxic loads. If one is very toxic with bromide, fluoride, Lyme and or heavy metals after a few days of taking Nascent Iodine you may after a few days of having more energy start to then feel lethargic. The lethargy is the body detoxing, stop the iodine for two or three days or when the detox lethargy goes away and start again with taking Nascent Iodine in the morning. You should feel that energy boost again for a few days and if you start to detox again and you feel lethargy, headache or another uncomfortable detox symptom stop for two or three days or until lethargy or detox symptoms go away. Some people do not want to start out taking a quarter drop of Nascent Iodine. In that case the other way I recommend starting Nascent Iodine is take one drop in water every fifth day for two weeks and see how you feel and react to Nascent Iodine. Then if all is well and you want to try more, then take one drop of Nascent Iodine in water every fourth day for another two weeks and as long as you feel good and do not have any uncomfortable detox symptoms or have not felt anything positive like extra energy, better focus, warming of cold hands and feet continue by taking one drop of Nascent Iodine in water every third day and then continue to shorten days between taking Nascent Iodine until you find how many drops and frequency works for you. I recommend this slow approach because Nascent Iodine is much more absorbable and faster acting than other forms of iodine such as in seaweed, seafood or other iodine supplements. Increase the number of drops of Nascent Iodine slowly over several weeks to be safe using only up to the maximum written on the label. Some people get good results with one drop of Nascent Iodine a week and others take anywhere between one and nine drops a day a few times a week depending on which Nascent Iodine they take. The three Nascent Iodine products I recommend have different amounts of iodine per drop so follow the directions on the label but start out slower and with less drops than the label recommends. We are all different in how much iodine we need. I stress going slow because of my own experience and others that I have introduced to Nascent Iodine. Some people get excited about their need for iodine or they start feeling positive results, or have cancer and iodine is anti-cancer, or want to bomb Lyme with iodine, and think that more iodine will give more results, but this is not always true and I have gotten reports back from people going through too much uncomfortable detox symptoms from taking too much iodine like a migraine headache, lethargy or night sweats. Iodine is a needed trace mineral not a needed macro-mineral. More is not better and can be actually counterproductive. There are people who take a half dropper of Nascent Iodine twice a week and some people put iodine on areas of their body that have cancer or tumors and report that it worked for them but I do not recommend that much iodine. I think too much iodine may be counterproductive in the long run. The body needs balance. My approach to immune health is to give the body the necessary foods and nutrients for health, not too much and not too little and at the same time eliminate the junk food and let the immune system take care of business. Make sure you are eating enough of a good quality salt on your food like Himalayan or Celtic Sea Salt. When we detox we need sufficient salt to transport toxins out of the body pathways in sweat, urine and bowel movements. Taking iodine without adequate salt is not recommended because not only does iodine push out the halogens bromide and fluoride but also the halogen chloride. Salt is sodium chloride so we must salt our food to our own taste to keep a balance of chloride to iodine in the body. That is why in 1924 the Morton Salt Company at the request of the United States Government put iodine in their salt to maintain that balance of iodine to chloride. Most people will only feel the energy boost and no detox symptoms, but there is a population that may detox for over one year. Other detox symptom can be a chemical smell on the breath or just bad breath and in the urine and sometimes the bottom of the feet can hurt. There is a urine test for bromide if you want to see how much bromide is being detoxed out of the body while taking iodine. If while dosing with iodine you experience night sweats or headache that is a sign you are taking too much iodine. Some people including myself when they first start taking Nascent Iodine may wake up in the middle of the night for an hour or two but this does not last for long, may be two or three days. Make sure your iodine dose is low at the start and you should be fine. This is just the body adjusting to the iodine. If you wake up at night, this happens to a few people when they first start taking iodine, just lay there and be calm, stay rested and you will still get your needed rest and know this waking up will pass soon and the iodine is working for your good. Nascent Iodine can also be administered by applying to the skin, but when applied to skin there is a delayed time of when the iodine becomes active and felt in the body as compared with oral dosing. We should also know what foods are goitrogenic which means they interfere with iodine uptake. The foods high in goitrogens are: soy and raw cruciferous vegetables. Gluten does not have goitrogens but it interferes with thyroid function. When cruciferous vegetables are cooked they lose most of their goitrogens making these vegetables safe and beneficial to eat. Cruciferous vegetables are broccoli, cabbage, cauliflower, kale, collards, mustard greens, bok choy, pak choi, tat soi, kamatsuna, mazuna, other asian greens, turnips, rutabaga, kohlrabi, brussel sprouts, radish, daikon radish, and broccoli raab. Broccoli sprouts do not have goitrogens. Millet has goitrogens and cooking does remove goitrogens in millet. Fermentation does not remove goitrogens from cabbage in sauerkraut. People can become deficient in iodine because of consuming large amounts of the goitrogenic foods soy and raw cruciferous vegetables and or being exposed to bromide and fluoride in the environment or in food and drinks. I used to make a 16 ounce raw vegetable juice about five days a week that consisted of one bunch of collards or one bunch of kale or one bunch of dandelion greens with about a half a cabbage, a few stalks of celery and the rest carrots. The amount of goitrogens I was getting from the bunch of collards or kale and cabbage was interfering with iodine absorption from foods and suppressing my thyroid, but I did not know it at the time. At that time I was also eating a lot of soy in the form of tofu, tempeh and gluten which also are iodine and thyroid suppressing. Eating an occasional raw kale salad may be okay for you but juicing raw cruciferous vegetables concentrates goitrogens. If you want to test if raw cruciferous vegetables are good for you I suggest trying to eat raw cruciferous vegetables plain without any dressing or seasoning or hiding it in a sugary fruit smoothie, let it stand by itself. If for instance you can eat a raw kale salad by itself and it tastes awesome to you then you are probably good to eat it. If it tastes nasty by itself then it is nasty for your body because you are tasting those goitrogens. When these goitrogenic substances are removed from the diet and iodine is supplemented, iodine stores in the body are replenished and many people can lower their dose of iodine. Nascent Iodine is the form of iodine that is most easily absorbed and can be most easily felt and thus each individual can determine their optimal dose. Foods that are high in iodine are number one seaweed and number two seafood. Foods containing lesser amounts of iodine are milk, yogurt, butter and eggs. Swimming in the ocean and breathing ocean air [especially air near ocean beaches with seaweed] is a way to get iodine. The reason dairy has iodine in the United States is because the udder of the cow, goat, or sheep is washed with iodine to clean the udder. This iodine is absorbed through the skin of the animal and ends up in the milk. Chicken eggs have iodine because iodine in the form of kelp is added to chicken feed, but still these farm foods may still be lacking in sufficient iodine for good health. Some people say they will just eat more iodine containing foods like seaweed or take a capsule of kelp, BUT if you have Lyme you owe it to yourself to try Nascent Iodine because of the profound effect Nascent Iodine can have on assisting the immune system in defeating Lyme and Lyme coinfections. Bromide and fluoride are two halogens that if the body does not have sufficient iodine, then bromide and fluoride will take iodine's place and wreak havoc in the body. Bromide is used in the following products, non organic flour and breads, in some vegetable oils, some sodas, in some farmed fish ponds, some cosmetics, some hair dyes, in fire retardant clothes, fire retardant furniture, fire retardant carpets, fire retardant drapes and curtains, new car smell is bromide off gassing, [it can take three years for bromide to finish off gassing from a new car], bromide is used as an agricultural pesticide, bromides are use in some pools and spas, bromide is used to poison rats, bromide is used in some municipal drinking water and in gasoline. Fluoride another halogen that interferes with iodine is in some municipal drinking water, some bottled water has added fluoride, some tooth paste, on some shaving blades, on some dental floss, some mouth washes, fluoride is in Teflon products use for waterproofing coats, gloves, boots, hats, in some lubricants, , in some ski wax and some fishing line. We need to protect ourselves from bromide, fluoride and heavy metals by making sure we are getting adequate iodine and staying away from exposure to bromide and fluoride. Everyone is different in how much iodine they need and what source of iodine they consume. One person may do well with Nascent Iodine, another with Lugols solution, another with Idoral, another with a supplement of potassium iodide and another eating seaweed and seafood. Once iodine stores are restored in the body and because iodine is recycled by the body and if one stays away from goitrogens and exposure to environmental bromides and fluorides then supplementation may be reduced. It is a good idea not to take iodine every day because the body could get too much of a good thing. Just like you would not eat your favorite food every day because you would get tired of it and that is the body saying we had enough of the nutrients in this food let's eat something else. I still want to stress and I think the easiest way for most people to self-dose iodine is with Nascent Iodine because it is so easy for most people to feel the effects of Nascent Iodine because most people after they have been taking Nascent Iodine for a while are able to feel when they need it and when they have taken too much. Usually people take it by how their energy level feels. If they lack energy they know they need iodine. If they take a little too much iodine they feel edgy or sometimes they call it feeling a little wired similar to drinking too much caffeine. Nascent Iodine may be better for some people because they have digestion that may be compromised and not able to absorb iodine sufficiently from food. Nascent Iodine is very easy to absorb and is recognized rapidly and easily by the thyroid. Once a person's iodine stores in the body are sufficient they may be able to maintain sufficient iodine through diet alone. The Australian government in 2009 has mandated iodized salt be added to the bread because the Australian government recognized that the population needs iodine for a healthy thyroid and for the development of infant's brain and nervous system during pregnancy and after pregnancy. I do not recommend iodized salt as the best source of iodine at least the iodized salt that I know of available in the United States because that iodized salt is a low quality salt and is mixed with anticaking agents.

The Japanese eat a lot of seaweed and seafood which amounts to about 1mg. to 3mg of iodine a day from their diet. Reference: https://www.ncbi.nlm.nih.gov/pmc/articles/PMC3204293/ Research shows that the iodine Japanese get in their diet negates the goitrogens found in fermented Japanese soy products. I am not recommending fermented soy products, though I do like natto for its high Vitamin K2 and probiotics, I just thought this is a good piece of information to show what iodine does as a nutrient with goitrogens from Japanese feremented soy. Many people say that Japanese fermented soy products are

healthy, I just do not have enough personal experience with the other Japanese fermented soy products as good or bad. I am just not a fan of soy because of the high phytoestrogens in soy and how phytoestrogens can weaken the immune system. This research did not show if iodine had any effect on the phytoestrogens in the fermented soy. Some other interesting information is that in Japan where the average person consumes approximately 1mg. to 3mg of iodine each day from seafood and seaweed is that Japan has on average 11 reported cases of Lyme each year.
Reference:
http://idsc.nih.go.jp/iasr/32/378/tpc378.html
https://wwwnc.cdc.gov/eid/article/20/8/13-1761_article#r6 whereas in the United States there are between 23,000 and 29,000 cases of Lyme reported each year.
Reference:
https://www.cdc.gov/lyme/stats/tables.html

The United States government estimates that the average person in the United States gets each day between 138mcg and 353mcg of iodine from food, which does not include supplementation with iodized salt or iodine containing dietary supplements. The average person in the United States gets eight times less iodine each day than the average person in Japan. Reference: http://ods.od.nih.gov/factsheets/IodineHealthProfessional/ The United States also consumes the most sugar per person in the world which is more than twice the amount of sugar the Japanese consume per person. There is more information on sugar in the Why Eliminate Sugar chapter. Two good books on iodine are 'Iodine Why You Need It Why You Can't Live Without' It by David Brownstein M.D. and 'The Iodine Crisis What You Don't Know About Iodine Can Wreck Your Life' by Lynne Farrow.

Chapter 16
Salt

Salt food to your personal taste is the most important rule with salt or any other food. Sodium is a necessary mineral for the body and salt contains many trace minerals. Salt has a bad rap in some circles as being a culprit for high blood pressure. It's usually not the salt, it's usually the sugar causing the high blood pressure. I know that salt can make the blood pressure go high and if that is the case I would suggest quitting sugar and salt. Then when blood pressure is stabilized, start adding salt to the diet and closely monitor blood pressure for any abnormal rise in blood pressure. We need salt to digest out food properly. Salt transports nutrients though the body. Salt helps the body detox by transporting toxins through detox pathways like sweat, urine and bowel movements, salt brings out the flavor in foods, salt kills pathogens, salt can be used as a bacteria killing toothpaste or mouth wash, gargle with salt water for a

sore throat, put salt water in a netti pot for a head cold, take a relaxing salt water bath, swim in the ocean and depending on where the salt comes from it can also contains other trace minerals besides sodium chloride. Use a good quality salt like Himalayan Salt or Celtic Sea Salt. Dr. David Brownstein in his book '
"Iodine Why You Need It Why You Can't Live Without It" says that salt is necessary for health and especially when supplementing with iodine. In 1924 the Morton Salt Company at the request of the United States Government put iodine in their salt. The Australian Government in 2009 mandated that bread in Australia have iodized salt. It has been known for a long time that salt and iodine go well together. Iodine and salt comes in a natural ocean package called seaweed.

Chapter 17
Warming And Cooling Foods
And Body Temperature

Most people suffering from chronic Lyme
have low body temperature. In the acute
stage of Lyme there can be a low grade
fever or a high fever. But the chronic Lyme
patient usually has a low body temperature.
In the iodine chapter it talks about how a
deficiency in iodine can cause low body
temperatures and when iodine becomes
sufficient in the body the body temperature
usually normalizes. There can be another
reason why the body temperature is low
and that can be a result of eating cooling
foods. To help restore normal body
temperatures we must look at the warming
and cooling foods. It is very popular now to
make raw smoothies, raw vegetable juices,
raw fruit juices and eat plenty of vegetable
and fruit salads. Now eating raw vegetables
is good but if someone has a low body
temperature, too much eating of raw
vegetables and raw fruits may be too

cooling for the body and especially in the winter if you are in an area that gets cold temperatures. The cooling vegetables are lettuce, greens of all types like kale, cabbage, collards, spinach, mustards greens, broccoli, tomatoes, peppers, eggplant, cucumber, zucchini, and yellow squash. When these vegetables are eaten raw they are more cooling than when cooked. Green tea is a powerful immune enhancing super food but is cooling to the body and may not be the right choice for someone with low body temperature. Try ginger, clove, cardamom, fennel or rosemary tea for a warming to the body tea. Black pepper is a warming spice we put on food. Oils high in polyunsaturated fats PUFAs like corn oil, canola oil, safflower oil, sesame oil, sunflower oil, peanut oil, soy oil, cotton seed oil, refined palm oil, grapeseed oil, flax oil, rice bran oil and almond oil and other nut oils are cooling to the body and they are high in omega 6 oils to omega 3 oils and this high ratio of omega 6 oils can suppress the immune system. These oils also become rancid easily. It is suspected that these PUFAs oils store in the body and can become rancid in the body. Chickens fed flax meal show rancid oil in their meat after they are butchered. To help warm the body temperature to normal it is best to eat foods like eggs, beef, bison, liver, goat, lamb, chicken, turkey and fish. Cook these meats in butter, ghee, coconut oil, olive oil or boil or pressure cook in water and then make a soup from the broth. Coconut oil is known to break up Lyme biofilms in the body. Other warming foods are root vegetables like beets, carrots, parsnips, turnip root, rutabagas, daikon radish root, other radish root, onions, garlic, and sweet potatoes. Cooking the cooling vegetables will make them less cooling. Sweet fruits are cooling. Rule of thumb is above ground vegetables are cooling and below ground vegetables are warming except for potatoes which are neutral and winter squash are warming. Have you ever noticed how we like raw vegetables and salads in the hot summer and less raw vegetables in the winter? That is because raw vegetables help cool the body and cooked root vegetables help warm the body. We should not eat raw vegetable in the cold winter just because we think that is good. We should tune into our bodies needs at the present time. The key is to balance eating these warming and cooling foods on how your body temperature feels.

Chapter 18
Oils And Fats
The Good And The Bad

Best oils are: Olive oil, 100% grass fed butter, 100% grass fed ghee, coconut oil, red palm oil and avocado oil. Coconut oil has been found to break up Lyme biofilms in the body. The richest tasting and the most nutritious olive oils come from the middle east. The awful oils are margarine, hydrogenated oils, partially hydrogenated oils and trans fats which it looks like the FDA is making illegal/banning, but keep an eye out because they may still allow partially hydrogenated oil/trans fats in packaged foods which is very deceptive because the headlines may read trans fats banned but that may not be the whole truth and trans fats may still be allowed in packaged foods. Buyer beware read the package. The bad oils are corn oil, canola oil, soy oil, flax oil, [flax oil is high in phytoestrogens and thyroid suppressing goitrogens and flaxseed has three times more phytoestrogens than soybeans], safflower oil, cotton seed oil, grapeseed oil, refined palm oil, sun flower oil and rice bran oil. These oils are high in polyunsaturated fatty acids PUFAs that have a track record of causing inflammation in the body. Who needs more inflammation? Some research shows these PUFAs can remain in the body for years after consumption is stopped and these PUFAs can release from fatty tissue into the blood stream for years and cause problems like thyroid suppression. Be patient after stopping the consumption of these PUFAs knowing it make take years to eliminate them from the body. Fasting, intermittent fasting and never overeating are good ways to accelerate the removal of PUFAs from the body.

The good oils are 100% green grass fed cows butter, 100% green grass fed cow or yak ghee, olive oil, coconut oil, red palm oil and avocado oil. These oils nourish the body and support the immune system.

Chapter 19
Turmeric More Than A Superfood

Richard Horowitz MD a holistic Lyme specialist says turmeric addresses Lyme Borreliosis and Babesia inflammation in the body and that turmeric is antiparasitic. Richard Horowitz has written two lengthy books on Lyme disease, Why I Can't Get Better? Solving The Mystery Of Lyme And Chronic Disease and How Can I Get Better An Action Plan For Treating Lyme & Chronic Disease. Dr Richard Horowitz talks a lot about drugs for Lyme which I am not in agreement with, but his book is still worth a read. If we include turmeric in the diet it will reduce inflammation and assist the immune system in exterminating Lyme disease. For best absorption turmeric should be eaten with black pepper and some kind of fat like 100% grass fed raw butter, 100% grass fed ghee, olive oil, coconut oil, red palm oil or avocado oil.
Benefits of Turmeric
1.Turmeric is anti inflammatory.

2. Turmeric is a natural pain killer.
3. Turmeric is a potent antioxidant.
4.Turmeric protects DNA.
5. Turmeric detoxifies heavy metals.
6. Turmeric is good for clear smooth skin.
7. Turmeric is a digestive aid.
8. Turmeric reduces arthritis pain.
9. Turmeric is good for bone health.
10. Turmeric is good for inflammation in muscles.
11. Turmeric helps alleviate depression.
12. Turmeric can improve memory.
13. Turmeric can protect against Alzheimer's.
14. Turmeric helps prevent stroke.
15. Turmeric helps prevent epilepsy and seizures.
16. Turmeric fights ear infections.
17. Turmeric can help glaucoma and cataract.
18. Turmeric mouthwash for reducing plaque and bacteria.
19. Turmeric supports healthy lung function.

20. Turmeric supports healthy liver function.
21. Turmeric supports healthy gallbladder function.
22. Turmeric reduces cholesterol levels.
23. Turmeric is anti-diabetic.
24. Turmeric assists weight loss by improving metabolism.
25. Turmeric relaxes blood vessels.
26. Turmeric supports a healthy thyroid.
27. Turmeric helps with hormonal imbalances.

28. Turmeric is heart and cardiovascular healthy.
29. Turmeric supports healthy urinary tract.
20. Turmeric supports healthy kidneys.
21. Turmeric supports healthy digestion and elimination.
22. Turmeric helps fight infections.
23. Turmeric inhibits replication of some viruses.
24. Turmeric is anti-candida.
25. Turmeric is anti- cancer.
26. Turmeric supports healthy bones.

27. Turmeric helps maintain healthy blood flow in the brain.

28. Turmeric boosts immunity and promotes longevity.

29. Turmeric helps protect against carcinogens.

30. Turmeric helps protect against food pathogens.

31. Turmeric is anti-parasitic.

32. Turmeric chelates iron in the body which can be good if your iron is too high. https://www.ncbi.nlm.nih.gov/pmc/articles/PMC6414192/

Best to get a ferritin test which is a test that measures iron stores in the body to see how turmeric affects your ferritin score. It is actually a great idea to get a ferritin test anyway because if your iron is too high or too low this can affect the immune system. Most doctors test only for serum iron which is a measurement of iron in the blood. Serum iron tests are included in the common CBC Complete Blood Count, but the ferritin test score is more important than serum iron, and you may need to request it from your doctor. I wanted to see how turmeric affected my ferritin. I had a ferritin blood test and then started taking about one teaspoon a day of turmeric with meals. About one month later I had another ferritin test and my ferritin score dropped by twenty percent.

Chapter 20
Ginger
More Than A Super Food.

Ginger is a warming food. Many people with Lyme have low body temperature. Having a cup of ginger tea in the morning can help with the coldness that many people with Lyme experience. Ginger is also anti parasitic. Sushi / raw tuna in restaurants is served with raw ginger just in case there are any parasites in the raw tuna. Ginger is a very good digestive aid raw or cooked and having a cup of ginger tea in the morning will help with morning elimination and breakfast digestion as well as helping warm the body. Ginger tea is a go to for cold and flu in Ayurveda and Traditional Chinese Medicine. Ginger fights nausea, fungal infections, protects against stomach ulcers, can ease menstrual pains, may inhibit cancer, regulates blood sugar, can relieve joint and muscle pain, improves brain function and blocks bacterial infections. As a digestive aid, Confucius wrote as far back as 500 B.C. of never being without ginger when he ate. In De Materia Medica 77 A.D. by Pedanius Diosorides wrote that ginger warms and softens the stomach. Ginger was used by the Roman Empire for digestion. In the Revolutionary War ginger was part of the soldier's diet. In the United States early 20th century, ginger was named the herb of choice for digestive support. The 5th century Chinese sailors used ginger to prevent scurvy. Everyone can be frequently exposed to intestinal parasites and raw ginger should be a part of every ones diet to keep the gut free from parasites. I have about a teaspoon of cut up fresh raw ginger with meals a few times a week and ginger has made a big difference in digestion. If you are a green tea drinker and are experiencing low body temperature, you might want to try some ginger tea. Green tea is a powerful immune enhancing drink, but may be too cooling to have every day for someone with a cold constitution and having some ginger tea

once in a while might just be the warmth
you need.

Chapter 21
Green Tea For Super Immunity
And It's Necessary Companion

Green tea boosts the immune system.
Green tea supports against colds, bronchitis
and flu. Green tea is anti-inflammatory
suppressing joint pain from arthritis. Green
tea is associated with supporting the
cardiovascular system. Green tea supports
healthy brain function. Green tea is anti-
cancer. Drinking green tea can relieve
sunburn within a few hours. Green tea gives
the body energy. But green tea has one
problem and that is high fluoride. There is a
way to keep fluoride out of the body or
remove the fluoride from the green tea
after it gets into the body and that is with
iodine. If the body does not have adequate
iodine then fluoride will go into the
receptor sites that iodine should be in such
as the thyroid, breasts, salivary glands,
pancreas, cerebral spinal fluid, skin,
stomach, brain, thymus, and muscles.
Iodine has also been found in every cell in

the body. If the body has adequate iodine, fluoride will be pushed out of the body. The country of Japan is the second largest consumer of green tea after China but per capita the Japanese are the largest consumers of green tea. The Japanese currently have the longest lifespan with the average being 92 years as of the writing of this book. The Japanese get an average of 1mg. to 3mg. of iodine in their diet every day from [mostly seaweed] and seafood which is plenty of iodine to keep the fluoride from green tea and other sources from lodging in the body. Traditionally the Japanese have a very short brew time for green tea from 30 seconds up to 3 minutes. Brewing green tea for longer than 3 minutes may accumulate too much caffeine in the tea water for some people. If you want to eliminate most of the caffeine from green tea, brew it for fifteen minutes, throw out the brewed tea and make another cup of tea with the just brewed tea leaves. When I make green tea I bring water to boil, then let water cool for two minutes and then brew a loose leaf green tea for eight minutes. My green tea brew time gives the brew water a golden hue. Brew time is individual for everyone and the type of green tea being brewed.

Chapter 22
Brewer's Yeast / Nutritional Yeast

During World War II Brewer's Yeast was a ration in the Australian Army in a product called Vegemite and the English Army had a Brewer's Yeast ration product called Marmite. Brewer's Yeast provides B-Vitamins, protein and minerals. It was included in their ration's because it was discovered that the troops had more stamina, were healthier and their immune systems were stronger if they ate Brewer's Yeast. Brewer's Yeast is one of the richest sources of the B Vitamins except the base formula does not contain Vitamin B12 but is added to some Brewer's Yeast. Vitamin B12 is easily found in animal products like: liver, beef, lamb, goat, chicken, eggs and fish. To be specific Brewyer's Yeast is a by-product of the beer making process. Nutritional Yeast is grown on a medium of beets or grains. The name Brewyer's Yeast is used interchangeable to describe the by-product of the beer making process and what is really Nutritional Yeast. I like Lewis Labs Nutritional Yeast that used to be called Brewyer's Yeast, and it is gluten free. Brewer's Yeast and Nutritional Yeast products vary in flavor so you made need to try different brands to find one you like and one that is gluten free. Nutritional Yeast is similar to Brewyer's Yeast in that they are made from the same yeast and they both have a good amount of B-Vitamins, protein and minerals. If you like neither Brewyer's Yeast or Nutritional Yeast, I recommend taking a B-Complex Vitamin to assist the immune system. Pure Synergy makes a Super B-Complex made with organic ingredients.

Chapter 23
Whey Protein

Whey Protein is the gold standard in protein. Whey Protein is a complete protein containing the nine essential amino acids. Whey Protein is used by athletes, body builders and fitness buffs because of the ability for Whey Protein to rapidly feed and repair muscle. If you exercise to hard or too much and feel soreness in the muscle from exercise, Whey Protein has such a high and good supply of protein that it can give the body what it needs to rapidly repair the muscle and relieve the soreness. Along with rebuilding muscle, whey protein contains bovine immunoglobulins that are similar to human immunoglobulins that support the immune system. Immunoglobulins are antibodies that identify and destroy foreign invaders like bacteria, parasites and viruses. Whey Protein has cysteine and glutamate which are precursors of glutathione which is a powerful antioxidant that detoxifies the body. Avoid Whey Protein Isolates and

Hydrolyzed Whey Protein because they have undergone too much processing. Whey Protein Concentrate is what you want. I like the brands WheyCool Whey Protein unflavored and Source Classic Organic Whey Protein unflavored. Both of these Whey Proteins are 100% grass fed, which means the cows are never fed grains. Whey Protein is also very high in lysine to lower arginine which makes this food a virus fighter too!

Chapter 24
Liver

Before multivitamin mineral tablets and capsules there was and still is the multivitamin mineral food beef and chicken liver. Liver is a concentrated source of highly available vitamins and minerals. The liver does not accumulate toxins as some think but filters and moves them out of the liver to other pathways to be eliminated by the body. Beef and chicken liver are nutrient rich meats and traditional were eaten once a week or once every other week as a nutrient boost. Liver is high in Vitamin A, B-Vitamins, selenium, copper and iron. Beef liver also has an awesome Vitamin K2 profile: MK4-MK6-MK7-MK8-MK9-MK10-MK11-MK12-MK13, try and find that in a vitamin pill. Do not eat liver more than once a week and only eat liver to your taste. What I mean by that is liver must taste good to you. That is the bodies way of saying I need what is in this food. Do not eat liver or any food that does not taste good to you just because you think it is good for you. Your taste buds are wise. Do not take desiccated liver tablets; they are made from raw dehydrated liver. Meat should always be cooked until there is no sign of red blood. Red blood can contain disease from the animal. When meat is fully cooked any disease will be destroyed. Liver contains a lot or iron. If you ate liver every day you would get too much iron. If you are anemic then you could eat liver more until you build your iron stores. My grandmother was diagnosed with anemia which is low iron. Liver was the go to medicine for anemia / low iron in her day. Her doctor told her to eat liver five days a week until she regained her strength and then eat liver no more than once a week. In my family we traditional ate liver once a week as did many other families' of that era. You should get your ferritin checked once a year if eating liver because of the high iron content in liver. A ferritin test shows how much iron is stored in the body. The ferritin test is different than the serum iron test which is included in a CBC Complete Blood Count test. The serum iron test shows iron in the blood only, not what is stored in the body. I had read that turmeric is a chelator of iron stores in the body. I did an experiment on myself. I had my ferritin checked and then added about a teaspoon a day of turmeric to my diet. I then had my ferritin checked about one month later and the lab test showed a twenty percent reduction in ferritin.

Chapter 25
Bone Broth

Bone broth traditionally was eaten only once a week. Bone broth is a potent concentration of highly absorbable minerals and collagen. Traditionally made from meat, cartilage and bones of beef or chicken and root and leaf vegetables. One can also use goat, lamb, turkey, duck and fish to make a bone broth soup. In my family we traditionally had meat bone broth with vegetables once a week. Bone broth can be high in collagen depending on what part of the animal is used to make the broth. Bone broth has become very popular. Traditional in my family my grandmother and mother would make a meat, bone and vegetable soup and we ate that soup one day a week. The caution that I raise is that chicken feet and their combs contain a lot of collagen as does beef marrow and knuckle bones. Collagen has a high arginine to lysine ratio. A balanced amount of collagen can be good but caution should be observed when eating high collagen soups too frequently. High arginine to low lysine ratio in the diet is known to feed viruses in the body. I was at one time eating a diet much higher in arginine and lower in lysine and I then personally experienced the virus Herpes Zoster which is Shingles which comes from the Chicken Pox virus. I personally came to this knowledge about the high arginine to low lysine ratio from getting skin manifestations of Shingles. I had a diet high in nut butter and unbeknown to me at that time is that nuts have a ratio that is high in arginine and low in lysine. I went to the Doctor after having what I thought were just insect bites on my head but they did not go away. The Doctor said I had shingles and said I got there too late for treatment but she prescribed a drug anyway. I do not remember the name of the drug but it cost $300.00 plus dollars for one bottle. I took this medicine for two days but it made me feel worse. While I was taking this medicine I got onto the internet and searched for natural cures for shingles. I came across information about how high arginine to low lysine in the diet feeds the herpes virus but high lysine to low arginine ratio prevents the virus from replicating. Since I like the nutrition approach to health, I stopped taking the drug and got some lysine and took 500mg of lysine with water before meals three times a day and stopped eating nuts and other high arginine to low lysine foods. Some recommendations are to take 1000mg of lysine with water before a meal, three times a day when fighting a herpes virus. I looked at food charts and made sure my diet was high lysine to low arginine. In three days I could feel the virus had been arrested and in three weeks the skin inflammation was gone and the [nerve pain / postherpetic neuralgia] was 99.9 percent better and eventually went away not too much later. My second outbreak was when I started eating chocolate which I had not done for many years and did not know chocolate was high in arginine. I got a rash on my side and thought it maybe poison ivy or shingles. I used to get poison ivy rash when I was in grammar school but not as an adult. I went to the Doctor for a diagnosis and he said it was shingles. He said he would give me a prescription but I said no thanks and told him my story the last time I had shingles and had success with taking lysine and restricting arginine. He was a little defensive at first, but said that lysine does work for some people. As we continued our conversation about lysine and arginine I said that I suspected that a high lysine to lower arginine diet would suppress many more viruses and he looked at me and said he agreed. I then thought to myself that this fact is medically known but hidden for the sake of making money with drugs and other medical therapies. The older Merck Pharmaceutical manuals have a lot of information on vitamins, minerals and other natural supplements and disease. Now this time instead of taking lysine I wanted to see if the rash would go away by diet along. I stopped eating chocolate and my diet is otherwise high in lysine ratio to low in arginine because I usually eat dairy, meat or fish three times a day and these protein foods are high in lysine and lower in arginine with dairy having the highest lysine to lowest arginine ratio . The rash went away without supplementing with lysine. The third time I had a herpes virus manifestation was from eating a high collagen chicken broth. I knew that collagen was high in arginine to lower lysine but wanted to see if it would manifest herpes virus in me. I wanted to make the chicken broth highly concentrated with collagen so I only used one pint of water for a whole chicken in the pressure cooker and the chicken still had the feet attached and chicken feet are very high in collagen. After about a week of having this high collagen chicken broth every day, I started to develop a manifestation of the herpes virus. I immediately stopped eating the high collagen chicken broth and the herpes virus symptoms went away. I believe that more lysine in the diet to arginine is important for the suppression of viruses and for a more robust immune system. Before I knew this information about viruses and higher lysine to lower arginine ratio, my mother suffered from shingles for about 13 years before she died. She was taking prescriptions for shingles and different therapies from doctors for shingles for about 13 years. Had I only know at that time what I know now she could have been on the way to being better in 13 days. Higher lysine to lower arginine is not the only factor to suppress viruses, because just taking lysine has not worked for everyone because there is much more to nutrition than one nutrient. No one nutrient is Lord of all, but I believe and research shows, higher lysine to lower arginine is a crucial part of health. Collagen is very high in the amino acid arginine. We want to watch our arginine to lysine ration because if we get more arginine than lysine it can feed viruses in the body and weaken the immune system. That is why I believe traditionally we only ate bone broth once a week. If bone broth is made low in collagen or without collagen than it can be eaten more than one day a week. I like to eat soup a few times a week, but my soup is very low in collagen. Collagen comes from animal cartilage, skin and marrow. Chicken feet are high in collagen too. Chicken combs contain hyaluronic acid. Some people eat a lot of high collagen bone broth and collagen supplements and seem to be healthy but I would still recommend anyone suffering from Lyme or other disease to be mindful of their lysine to arginine ratio in their diet.

Chapter 26
Dr. Zhang Protocol

Dr. Zhang developed an herbal protocol that has been used in China to treat a similar to Lyme spirochete. His protocol consists of Allicin in one capsule, Artemisiae in another capsule and Circulation P in another capsule. Dr. Zhang developed other herbal products for Lyme but these three are the main ones. The Allicin capsule is from garlic. I asked Dr. Zhang if I could just eat garlic instead of taking his Allicin capsules. Dr. Zhang said "There are TWO GARLIC BULBS worth of allicin in one Allicin capsule." The Allicin capsule exterminates Lyme Borellia burgdorferi, the Artemisiae exterminates Babesia and bursts Lyme Borrella cysts. Artemisiae is also used to exterminate the Malaria parasite and the Circulation P is a mix of herbs that increases the bodies circulation to help deliver the Allicin and Artemisiae and help with sluggish circulation. Many people with Lyme suffer from sluggish circulation. A prescription is not needed for Dr. Zhang's herbs and can be ordered online with a search for Dr. Zhang Lyme protocol or at www.drrons.com. Dr Zhang recommends taking the herbs for six months. It is suspected that Lyme may stay dormant or suppressed in the body for possibly years and then manifest under a stressful event or weakened immune system. I took Dr. Zhang's herbs for two months and I felt it was enough and felt so much better and felt that the Lyme was gone and also felt if I kept taking the herbs for much longer it would throw my body out of balance. I found Dr. Zhang's herbal protocol to be very good for removing my acute case of Lyme. Years later I got Lyme again and Dr. Zhang's herbal protocol did not work for me at that time. Many people have benefited from Dr. Zhang's herbal protocol. Dr. Zhang has a book "Lymes Disease and Modern Chinese Medicine" and in this book Dr. Zhang explains his protocol.

Chapter 27
Wormwood / Artemisia absinthium

As mentioned in Dr. Zhang's Lyme Protocol, there is a capsule called Artemisiae which is Artemisia. Wormwood is the common name and latin name is Artemisia absinthium and can be purchased in health food stores or online and is available organic. Artemisia is used effectively for malaria in many countries. A two day dose of Artemisia for malaria is given and is usually sufficient. Artemisia is effective at treating the Lyme coinfection Babesia and breaking apart Lyme Borrelia cysts. Artemisia will also eliminate intestinal parasites. Some people will pulse taking Artemisia two days on and between five and seven days off and then take Artemisia for another two days doing this for two months because some research shows absorption of Artemisia into the bloodstream slows after taking it for two days. Dr. Zhang does not recommend pulsing of Artemisiae.

Chapter 28
Cholesterol And Why You Need It

Cholesterol is needed for immune health and total cholesterol under 200 can be downright dangerous. LDL is usually called bad cholesterol but this is not always true. LDL cholesterol can be bad but it can also be very good! There is a blood test that can show if the LDL is bad or good. The test is called a Lipoprotein Particle Test. This test shows the particle size for the LDL cholesterol. If the LDL particles are large they are protective to the cardiovascular system and that is good. If the LDL particles are small then they are oxidized and could be trouble for cardiovascular system and this is bad. The Lipoprotein Particle Test gives a score for oxidized LDL with a range scale. Research shows that people who have total cholesterol 220 to 260 have fewer infections and lower rates of cancer than those who have cholesterol between 100 and 199! Low cholesterol is also linked to Alzheimer's because the brain needs cholesterol to function properly and for good cognition. Cholesterol is brain food. Then why do doctors and even most natural health professionals recommend total cholesterol between 100 and 199. The reason is the FDA recommends those numbers and if a doctor or health professional tells their patients that cholesterol at 220 and above is healthy and that person suffered a heart attack or stroke then a slick lawyer and an angry patient or family could sue the doctor or health professional for mal practice. Statin drugs that lower cholesterol is a billion dollar industry and when a person may get Alzheimer's because their brain is low on cholesterol [cholesterol is food for the brain] there are Alzheimer drugs that make for another billion dollar industry and so the snowball grows. Get the picture? Statin drugs also deplete the body of COQ10 and vitamin K2 of which adequate levels are important for cardiovascular health.

To get more accurate information of cardio health get the blood LDL particle size test,

C-Reactive Protein Cardiac, Myeloperoxidase, Homocysteine and Fibrinogen Activity. These blood tests can show regardless of cholesterol numbers if there is inflammation in the cardiovascular system. A Calcium Scan will show if you have any calcium building up on your arteries and if so vitamin K2 can help reduce the calcium building up on arteries and other soft tissue. The best sources of Vitamin K2 are natto and butter from cows eating rapidly growing green grass. I have taken supplement pills of Vitamin K2 and have found that natto and butter from cows eating rapidly growing green grass are much better. You can't beat the real thing. Many people take high doses of vitamin D3 but neglect the vitamin K2 and high doses of vitamin D3 without vitamin K2 can cause calcification in the arteries and other soft tissue. Vitamin K2 is the truck driver for calcium bringing it to where it belongs in the body. Some people recommend for every 1000 IU of vitamin D one should take 100mcg of vitamin K2. I personally do not supplement with Vitamin D3 or recommend taking Vitamin D3. I get Vitamin D from food and I do work outside for my job but I wear a long sleeved shirt, long pants and sun hat so not get too much sun. My shirt is thin so maybe I get some Vitamin D through my thin shirt from the sun. I get plenty of Vitamin K2 from 100% green grass fed cows butter and natto. The highest MK4 source of Vitamin K2 is from butter from cows eating rapidly growing green grass. I would also put grass fed raw cows butter in the class of an immune boosting superfood. The highest MK10 source of Vitamin K2 is from natto. Natto is usually made from soybeans but can easily be made with chickpeas or black beans using the yogurt setting on the Instant Pot. There is more to the Vitamin D story especially for someone with Lyme or another chronic disease or anyone for that matter. The common recommended blood test for Vitamin D is 25HD or more accurately called 25-hydroxyl-vitamin D precursor. This measures the amount of precursor to make Vitamin D, not the active

Vitamin D in the body. The test that needs to compliment 25HD is the 1,25HD or more accurately called 1,25-dihydroxy-calcitriol-vitamin D which is the active Vitamin D. The active secosteroid hormone 1,25-dihydroxy-calcitriol-vitamin D can be normal while the 25-hydroxyl-vitamin D precursor is low. If anyone relies on Vitamin D dosing because of a low 25-hydroxyl-vitamin D precursor score but unknowingly is normal or high in active 1,25-dihydroxy-calcitriol-vitamin D they could make their immune system weaker by taking Vitamin D. Both Vitamin D tests should be done to get a better evaluation of Vitamin D status. I myself test low on the Vitamin D precursor test but I am in the normal range for active Vitamin D and I do not supplement with Vitamin D. I suspect that not everyone converts Vitamin D precursor to active Vitamin D the same. I believe it is erroneous to dose Vitamin D from results on a Vitamin D precursor test without knowing the active Vitamin D. See the chapter on Vitamin D for more information.

Cholesterol is needed for healthy hormones. From cholesterol comes the hormones pregnenolone, DHEA, progesterone, androstenediol, androstenedione, cortisol, aldosterone, testosterone, estrone, estradiol, estriol and more. If you want healthy hormones you need sufficient cholesterol. The body also makes over sixty steroids from cholesterol. Total cholesterol between 220 and 260 is needed for a strong robust immune system and through blood tests you can get information on your cardio vascular system and make your own educated decisions. Some research shows that even higher cholesterol numbers are healthy too. My last total cholesterol was 220 but I had total cholesterol of 330 for a while and my LDL particles were still the large protective LDL particles, my HDL was high and my other cardiovascular blood tests: C-Reactive Protein Cardiac, Myeloperoxidase, Homocysteine and Fibrinogen Activity showed no inflammation in the cardio vascular system. I usually do these blood tests once a year. What moved my cholesterol from 330 to 220 was the addition of about four ounces a day of red wine before dinner. I did not start drinking wine for cholesterol reasons, but that is what I noticed on my cholesterol numbers when the only change I made was the wine. Total cholesterol is not a valid marker to determine heart health.

Other cardio vascular blood test markers need to be factored into the equation. Becoming over stressed either physically, mentally, fear, constant worry, lack of exercise, eating junk foods, non-organic food, sugar, soy and gluten are some of the worst things for the heart.

Chapter 29
Take Care Of Your Teeth

Bacteria can build up in the mouth and cause the immune system unneeded stress. Food can get caught between the teeth causing bacteria to form. If we brush and floss we can keep bacteria levels in the mouth under control and relieve the immune system to fight in other areas of the body. If you have mercury amalgam fillings get them out by a dentist who knows what he is doing with mercury amalgam fillings removal and takes precautions so you don't swallow or breathe any mercury during removal and the dentist can assist you with detox strategies for mercury. Root canals can also harbor bacteria so it may be better to lose the tooth than have to put unneeded stress on immune system with the bacteria under the root canal. Drink raw milk from A2 cows, goats or sheep that are 100% green pasture grass and hay fed and eat their raw butter and cheese, because they are superior for dental and bone health than pasteurized dairy. I am not against pasteurized dairy, both are good and have their place. There are nutrients that are available from raw dairy that cannot be had with pasteurized dairy and there are nutrients from pasteurized dairy that cannot be had with raw dairy so it is beneficial to eat both. Most cheese and yogurt are pasteurized. I highly recommend rinsing the mouth with grass fed A2 cows raw milk, goat or sheep milk before eating and drinking and after eating and drinking. Even if you cannot drink and digest milk, this rinsing of the mouth with raw milk will do wonders for your teeth and health without digestive upset. The teeth love raw milk. Raw milk is absorbed by the teeth and raw milk creates beneficial flora in the mouth. Raw dairy can regenerate the teeth. Read the chapter on dairy for more information. Natto is another superfood that can benefit the teeth because Natto is high in Vitamin K2, and K2 is known to strengthen teeth and bones by bringing calcium to the teeth and bones.

Chapter 30
Paleo Diet Is It For You

At the writing of this book the Paleo Diet based on The Hunter Gatherer Diet has become extremely popular with some folks. I am not here to argue, if you like the Paleo Diet and it is working for you, that is good. I want to share some general research on Hunter Gatherers. This research is for living current Hunter Gatherers: Researchers Gurven and Kaplan have estimated that around 57% of hunter gathers reach the age of 15. Of those that reach 15 years of age, 64% continue to live to or past the age of 45. This places there life expectancy between 21 and 37 years. They further estimate that 70% of deaths are due to diseases of some kind, 20% of deaths come from violence or accidents and 10% are due to degenerative diseases. I think the Paleo Diet can be dangerous because so many cultures of the world have survived for thousands of years on beans, grains, meats and dairy but the hunter gatherer

Paleo Man is dead. The addition of beans and grains provided the necessary energy for these cultures to work hard long days. The Paleo Diet is unsustainable. The carbohydrates in beans and grains provide energy. I know people on the Paleo Diet that have told me they do not have the same energy as they did when eating beans and grains. Carbohydrates from beans and grains feed the immune system. Without beans and grains the immune system will suffer.

I personally feel the best way with the most benefits to get keto is with fasting from solid food. I like doing a yearly vegetable broth fast and during the rest of the year skip the last meal of the day now and then, never over eat and never snack between meals and or fast more whenever I feel the need. Fasting does things for the body that no other modality can do. Fasting can be difficult because we get physically weak when we fast, but the fast is only temporary and well worth the effort. The longest lived people at the time of this book being written are the Japanese with the average lifespan of 92. The Japanese eat white rice every day. I network with multitudes of people on diet. What I have found out with those that say they do the Paleo Diet is that most are not 100% Paleo. They do incorporate beans and grains into their diet based on desire. What else I have found out is that many peoples main grain for eating is wheat. When someone stops or lowers their intake of wheat/gluten/glue [latin name for glue is gluten] they will feel better. Gluten can impair digestion, cause leaky gut, destroy the villi in the small intestine, stick on the gut for years, cause constipation, cause brain fog, joint pain, promote allergies, cause enlarged heart and interfere with the thyroid. Eat the good grains: white rice, buckwheat, oats, amaranth, quinoa and add in beans. Grains and beans eaten together make for a more complete protein when they are eaten together. Beans have more minerals than grains. Beans are alkaline and grains are acid. Grains and beans support a healthy immune system. The longest lived Japanese people are a testament to that fact. Plus grains and beans need to be prepared a certain way to make them healthy to eat. The Japanese eat white rice because brown rice contains a lot of anti-nutrients called phytates. Phytates are anti-nutrients that bind with good minerals in the gut preventing absorption and tax the digestive system. White rice also has the least amount of anti-nutrients than any other grain. All grains and beans have anti-nutrients and that is the problem with grains and beans, but the way we prepare grains and beans is most important because we must do this in a way that removes the problem causing anti-nutrients. All grains and beans except white rice should be soaked in water overnight and throw away the soak water and rinse the grains and beans. If a pressure cooker is used, grains and beans only need to be rinsed and do not need to be soaked overnight because a pressure cooker will remove anti-nutrients and preserve good nutrients. Remove the pressure cooker water from beans and rinse the beans well. Complex carbs from good grains and beans with anti-nutrients removed support a healthy immune system. I think a lot of problems that people have with grains and beans are due to not preparing and cooking them properly to remove ant-nutrients and also eating packaged foods that have grains and beans that have not been properly prepared to remove anti-nutrients. Commercially canned beans are cooked in a pressure cooker so the anti-nutrients have been removed, just make sure to throw out the water in the can of beans and then rinse the beans. Another benefit to beans is that some beans have a higher lysine and lower arginine ratio such as black turtle beans, red kidney beans, pinto beans, navy beans and great northern beans. Grains have a higher arginine to lower lysine ratio.

I do not recommend brown rice even after going through soaking or pressure cooking because there are still too many anti-nutrients in brown rice. The longest lived

people as of the writing of this book are the
Japanese and they eat white rice.

Chapter 31
Fasting

Over eating is a strain on the immune system. It is always better to under eat a little than to over eat a little. When we fill our bellies with more food than we need, the body needs to put energy into moving the excess unneeded food through the body, or storing it as fat and thus leaving less energy for other systems of the body like the immune system. Excess food becomes a toxin instead of a benefit. It is always best to eat just enough to satisfy our hunger or a little bit less. If we stop eating a little bit before we are satisfied, usually we will be satisfied about twenty to thirty minutes later. If each meal is balanced with protein, complex carbohydrates and fat it is much easier to not overeat. Learn which combination of good foods satisfies your hunger. Having two different types of animal proteins with a meal may satisfy your hunger better, such as meat with cheese or egg and cheese.

Fasting is a good way to renew the immune system and the whole body. If you are new to fasting, an easy way to start fasting is with intermittent fasting. That is when one skips one or two meals a day. The body likes to fast/cleanse, renew and rebuild at night. If we go to bed with a full stomach we hinder the body's ability for rejuvenation. Skipping one meal a day is the easiest way to start getting the benefits of fasting. I recommend skipping the last meal of the day because then the belly is sure to be empty when going to sleep. It is best to get to sleep by 9 or 10 o'clock. Our bodies are hooked up with where the sun is in the sky. The body is going to cleanse and rebuild according to sun time not our time. We want our bellies empty before 9 o'clock. The body wants to do a mini fast every night. That is why the first meal in the morning is called break fast. Just doing intermittent fasting by skipping the last meal of the day once in a while will give the digestive system a longer rest and has been proven to renew the body and extend life.

When you have done intermittent fasting for a while you may want to try a one or two day fast. If you want to get even more benefits then do three days or more. Work your way up slowly increasing the days of the fast. Listen to your body because sometimes the body just tells us we need to fast with signs like diminished hunger or bloating, and listen to your body on when to brake the fast which will come with experience. If you say you are going to do a three day fast or a seven day fast, do not hold yourself to how many days you decided to fast. Just take each day one at a time and if you start feeling too weak or ill then break the fast. From experience you will learn when it is time to break the fast. During a fast even though we get physically weak, there are good things that are felt. There are positive things that happen to the body during the fast. The brain can operate much faster and clearer, the digestive system is quiet, there is a knowing that we are doing something good for the body, and the body is getting some much needed cleaning, rest and renewal. During the fast one is not always tired. I have experienced times during a fast where I had normal energy as if I was eating, but I learned that even though that I had normal energy during the fast I should not use that energy in physical activity. One time after a few days into a fast I was not tired and had normal energy and I did some physical work outside and it felt great but the next day I paid for it and was very tired and just laid on the couch most of the day. Now when I feel that normal energy during a fast I do not do any vigorous physical work, but save that energy for the body to use for the cleansing and renewal of the body. When fasting I do not recommend any physical exercise because the body's enzymes are leaving the digestive system and are eating up the garbage throughout the body, and we do not want to break down muscle tissue from exercise because the muscle will then be looking for food to rebuild what was torn down during exercise. We must conserve our energy during a fast to make it most successful and only walk a little bit or go for short errands to the store. Make sure you drink plenty of water and or vegetable broth during the fast. If you do just fine on just drinking water during the fast that is good. If you start to feel bad on a water fast then try making some cooked vegetable broth and just drink the broth and do not eat the vegetables. It is amazing how much easier the fast can be by drinking cooked vegetable broth during a fast. From my fasting experience the best is just water and or cooked vegetable broth, but you may be different. I have found that vegetable broth makes the fast a whole lot easier and actually fun for me as compared to a straight water fast. I do not recommend drinking fruit juice, sugared water or raw vegetable juice on a fast. People who drink fruit juice or sugared water run the risk of getting candida during the fast. There is a fast I do not recommend called the Master Cleanse, where lemon juice, water and maple syrup are mixed together. The maple syrup is a recipe for overgrowth candida.

What first inspired me to do a two week fast is the rejuvenation that takes place at the two week mark of rebooting the hormones. I had dabbled in fasting the most three days until one day I was getting a delivery of chicken manure for my organic vegetable farm and asked the truck driver how long do the farmers keep their egg laying chickens. He said once the chickens start laying eggs they keep them for one year because after that the hens slow down laying eggs, but he said some farmers will after one year of the hens laying, put their hens on a water fast for two weeks, and after the two week fast the hens lay eggs good for another year. I then thought, I got to try the two week fast. After a two week vegetable broth fast it took me about five days of eating very light, but once my digestive system got going I ate small meals from 6:30 in the morning every hour to 9:30 at night. If I did not eat every hour on the hour my stomach would hurt. After about two weeks of eating like this, the weight I had lost during the fast was back, and I returned to my normal three meals a day. It was probably the most fun I have ever had with food! I know I just said earlier in this chapter to have the belly empty before 9 o'clock and I just said when I returned to eating after my fast I was eating at 9:30 pm, but I was just going with what my body was telling me at that time and it felt right. My body was telling me what it needed and my digestive system was digesting food more efficiently and faster than I have ever experience before and after about two weeks of eating like this I went back to three meals a day with my last meal of the day around 6:30pm to 7:00pm. If you do not want to fast at least make sure you do not over eat or go to bed with a full stomach because over eating and going to bed with a full stomach will prevent the immune system and the rest of the body from working at its best. Digestion requires a lot of energy and the body prefers to have an empty stomach at night when sleeping. The body wants to fast and cleanse the body and repair when sleeping at night.

That is why the morning meal is called break fast. My longest fast so far has been two weeks but I know of people who have had successful fasts to forty days. I believe forty days is the longest anyone should fast. There is research that after forty days the body may break down the organs for food. The best way to break a fast for me and others that I know who fast often is with a soft or hard boiled or poached egg. Many books and other material that I have read on fasting recommend breaking a fast with fruit or vegetables, but myself and other fasters I know break their fasts with a soft or hard boiled or poached egg. I have tried breaking fasts with fruit or vegetables but fruit or vegetables do not break the fast, they just continue the fast. When it is time to break the fast the body is looking for protein and an easy to digest protein and an egg is very good protein and easy to digest. If I have been on a seven day or two week fast, when I break the fast I have just one egg for breakfast the first day and it may take me an hour to eat one egg because I want to feel how my stomach responds to the first food after a fast. The second day I will have one egg for breakfast and one egg for lunch. The third day I will have one egg for breakfast, one egg for lunch and one egg for dinner. The fourth day I will have one egg and a rice cake for breakfast, one egg and a rice cake for lunch, and one egg and a rice cake for dinner. By the fifth day my digestion is starting to wake up more and comeback strong but I just feel it out because I do not want to put too much food into my belly until it is ready. I would much rather under eat than over eat. Overeating would tax the digestive system before it is ready for a normal sized meal. When I feel my digestive system starting to really crank up I will add a little steak to the diet and I eat mostly steak, eggs, rice cakes with a little olive oil on the rice cakes and then add a little bit of pressure cooked or steamed vegetables like peas and greens. It usually takes me the same number of days to recover from the fast as how many days I have fasted and put the weight back on that

I lost during the fast. I use rice cakes because they are an easy to digest complex carb. When breaking a fast we always must go slow. We never want to eat our normal size meals when we break a fast because the stomach has shrunk and the digestive enzymes are not very active in the stomach for the first few days after breaking a fast because the enzymes have been other places in the body eating up toxins and damaged tissue. If someone ate a normal sized meal after a three day or more days fast, the normal sized meal would overload the digestive system and one would lose some of the benefits of the fast and it can feel very uncomfortable. Breaking the fast requires discipline and it is worth resisting the urge to eat too much when breaking the fast. The more days a person fasts, the more careful one needs to be when breaking the fast. You should get checked out by a doctor before you fast and or be monitored by a doctor or health professional while you are on a fast and when you break a fast if you are not comfortable fasting by yourself. Fasting is hard, but a fast can have very rewarding times during and after the fast. I like to think of fasting as being on Creators operating table. In the past when I would have a challenge in my stomach or intestines I would think, "Well I can go to the doctors and have them stick a periscope in my gut and get prescribed drugs or surgery or I can fast first and see what happens from a fast." I have always been glad I chose the fast.

My severe stomach bloating from gluten forced me to learn how to fast and lead me to the discovery that it was the gluten that made my stomach bloat. I have to say that fasting can be hard, but my fear of going to the doctor for invasive probes, prescription drugs and possible surgery was the strongest motivation that made me fast. A blessing in disguise. Now when I fast I am prepared for the uncomfortable parts of the fast, but I now know that the health rewards are well worth it.

There is a powerful cleansing and renewing of the body that happens during a fast, [that only fasting can accomplish.]

Chapter 32
Vitamin D Supplements
May Not Be Good For You

There is more to the Vitamin D story that is commonly told and especially for someone with Lyme or another chronic disease or anyone for that matter. The common recommended blood test for Vitamin D is 25HD or more accurately called 25-hydroxy-vitamin D precursor. This measures the amount of precursor in the body to make Vitamin D not the active Vitamin D. The 1,25-dihydroxy-calcitriol-vitamin D test measures the active form of Vitamin D which is produced in the liver and kidneys through the conversion of 25-hydroxy-vitamin D precursor. The common recommended test to evaluate adequate Vitamin D in the body is the 25-hydroxy-vitamin D precursor test. If the conversion of 25-hydroxy-vitamin D precursor to 1,25-dihydroxy-calcitriol-vitamin D works the same in everyone, than this would be an accurate test for everyone, but everyone does not convert 25 hydroxy-vitamin D precursor to 1,25-dihydroxy-calcitriol-vitamin D the same. The 25-hydroxy-vitamin D precursor score maybe useful for some people but not all and especially not for chronic Lyme or others with chronic diseases. The test that needs to compliment the 25-hydroxy-vitamin D test is the 1,25-dihydroxy-calcitriol-vitamin D which is the active Vitamin D. The 1,25-dihydroxy-calcitriol-vitamin D test is used when investigating a problem related to bone metabolism, parathyroid function, kidney failure and possible Vitamin D deficiency. The active secosteroid hormone 1,25-dihydroxy-calcitriol-vitamin D can be low, normal or high in some people and those with Lyme or others with chronic disease, and even in populations that are healthy, while the 25-hydroxy-vitamin D is low. If some people or those with Lyme or others with chronic disease relies only on a Vitamin D dosing amount because of a low 25-hydroxy-vitamin D precursor score but unknowingly have normal or high active

1,25-dihydroxy-calcitriol-vitamin D and they start supplementing with Vitamin D it could make 1,25-dihydroxy-calcitriol-vitamin D too high, overload the body with Vitamin D, draw excess calcium into the soft tissue, heart and kidneys, and make the immune system weaker. Both tests should be done to get a better evaluation of Vitamin D status and you should have this done by a knowledgeable doctor in this field.

Low serum 25-hydroxy-vitamin D precursor could be the body protecting itself from making too much Vitamin D and then bringing in too much calcium into the blood stream and thus causing calcification of the aortic valve of the heart, coronary arteries, and other soft tissue in the body. If someone takes Vitamin D without taking adequate Vitamin K2 it is a recipe for disaster causing calcification of the soft tissue because without adequate Vitamin K2 in the body Vitamin D can deposit calcium where it does not belong. A coronary calcium scan can detect and measure calcification [calcium containing plaque] in the arteries. I do not recommend taking supplemental Vitamin D3 but if you do take Vitamin D3 some people recommend taking Vitamin K2 at a ratio for each 1000 IU of Vitamin D3 take 100mcg. of Vitamin K2 to help prevent calcification of arteries and other soft tissue. Better yet eat natto as it is the highest food source of Vitamin K2 and is also probiotic. I have taken many different Vitamin K2 supplements and now eat natto, raw grass fed butter and raw milk for my main sources of Vitamin K2. These food sources are far superior to Vitamin K2 pill supplements. My 25-hydroxy-vitamin D score is low below 30 but my 1,25-dihydroxy-calcitriol-vitamin D is in the middle of the range and I do not take Vitamin D. I used to take Vitamin D and brought my 25-hydroxy-vitamin D score to give or take 50 ng/mL, but I stopped taking Vitamin D because my immune system is stronger when I do not take Vitamin D. If you want to supplement with Vitamin D I would recommend cod liver oil because it has a diverse array of vitamin D compounds along with high Vitamin A and omega 3 fatty acids. Cod liver oil was the go to supplement in the days before vitamin pills. The only cod liver oil I can recommend are Dropi Pure Icelandic Cod Liver Oil and Rosita Extra Virgin Cod Liver Oil because they are pure unadulterated cod liver oil. Many companies add synthetic Vitamin A and synthetic Vitamin D to their cod liver oil. Making cod liver oil is as simple as throwing cod livers into a bucket of water, the cod livers sink to the bottom of the bucket and in a few days the cod liver oil rises to the top and is scooped off the top of the water. Cod liver oil made this way many years ago was called grade A cod liver oil. After the cod liver oil was scooped off the top of the water, they took those same cod livers and made Grade B cod liver oil out of these same cod livers. Grade B cod liver oil was brown cloudy cod liver oil and was made by a machine that pressed the cod livers and then strained out most of the solids but is not pure oil because it contains some pressed liquefied meat from the cod liver which gives it the brown color.

It is important to note that Vitamin D3 is not really a vitamin but a steroid hormone. The majority of the Vitamin D3 steroid hormones in supplements are made from lanolin that comes from sheep wool and the other minor source is from Lichen. Lichens are a fungus that live symbiotically with algae or cyanobacteria. Are steroid hormones from sheep wool or fungus that would not be a part of a natural diet, be the best or even good for the human body? Vitamin D3 steroid hormone from lanolin made from sheep wool is also used as a rat poison. Vitamin D3 and calcium are mixed with bait blocks or bait pellets. The heart and kidneys are the target organs for the rodents. Mice and rats eat this Vitamin D3 calcium laced bait and within three to four days get hypercalcemia, which results in calcification of soft tissue, leading to cardiac arrest or kidney failure.

Reference:
https://www.ncbi.nlm.nih.gov/pmc/articles/PMC6122607/

Get a coronary calcium scan to see if you have calcification in the arteries. I do not take cod liver oil or supplement with Vitamin D, and when out in the sun I am covered most of the time with clothing [long sleeved shirt, pants and sun hat] and my active Vitamin D is normal. If you really think you must supplement with Vitamin D3, I would recommend no more than 400 to 600 IU per day for an adult and also take with that 100mcg of Vitamin K2. It is best to get both Vitamin D tests discussed here to see what are your active Vitamin D and your precursor Vitamin D scores.

Chapter 33
Vitamin C And
Intravenous Vitamin C

The first time I got Lymes disease I did a six week run of Doxycycline. While I was on Doxycycline the Lyme symptoms were suppressed but still quite evident. After I finished the six week run of Doxycycline the Lyme systems came back just as strong as before I started taking Doxycycline. I went back to the doctor for more Doxycycline but they said they would not give me anymore and recommended a local Lyme specialist doctor. I said I would make an appointment with this specialist doctor but I said I really needed more Doxycycline to suppress the symptoms until I had my appointment with the Lyme specialist. They gave me another prescription of Doxycycline. I made the appointment with the Lyme specialist and a few days later I was wondering what course of action they had for Lymes disease. I called the Lyme specialist and was told that antibiotics were given for Lymes disease.

After another day or so of thinking about getting more antibiotics I felt that was not the way to go for me. My condition was extreme mental fog, weakness, and night sweats that completely soaked my clothes. I felt that more antibiotics would just weaken my body more and not give me the cure. I prayed for an answer. I believe that our Creator is very interested in us, our life, and being well. One morning when I was coming out of sleep with completely sweat soaked shirt and pants these thoughts came into my mind, "Intravenous Vitamin C." I did not give those thoughts much credence. The next morning coming out of sleep with sweat soaked clothes the same thoughts came into my mind, "Intravenous Vitamin C." I still did not give those thoughts much credence. The third morning coming out of sleep with sweat soaked clothes the same thoughts came into my mind "Intravenous Vitamin C". This time I thought "I think God is trying to get a message across to me." I then called a well known biochemist chiropractor in town to ask him if he provided the service of Intravenous Vitamin C. The office staff told me no but gave me a phone number of a Doctor who did provide the service of Intravenous Vitamin C. I made an appointment for my first drip of Intravenous Vitamin C. This was the winter time and I was not working my normal seasonal job which is organic farming, organic lawns, and organic pest control for homes and landscapes. I decided to take a delivery job for the winter using my own vehicle. I would call dispatch in the morning and they would give me an address for a pick up and I would deliver the package. After delivering the package I would call dispatch again for another pickup and delivery. I started in New Jersey and a delivery day could take me to New York City, upstate New York and to the southern tip of New Jersey. The day of my appointment I decided to stop work to give myself enough time to make my appointment for the Intravenous Vitamin C. The day of my appointment came and I was apprehensive about having a needle stuck in my arm with a large dose of Vitamin C, and apprehensive about if I had really heard from God about doing this treatment. My first dose was to be 35 grams of Vitamin C. The doctor told me I should have two Vitamin C drips the first week, and then a Vitamin C drip every week for a total of ten Vitamin C drips. The doctor told me there was also some calcium and magnesium in the drip to balance the Vitamin C. The day came and I was delivering packages and watching my time. My appointment for the Vitamin C drip was in the evening. Towards the end of the day when time was getting close to stop delivering packages, I had a call to pick up a package and the delivery address was about two miles down the road from the office where I was to get the Intravenous Vitamin C. When I saw where I ended up about two miles down the road from the doctor's office, I knew for sure that God had orchestrated this event and God wanted me to have the Intravenous Vitamin C. I had my first Vitamin C drip on a Monday and did not feel any better. My next visit was Wednesday of the same week. When I woke up the next morning I felt better than I had felt since I got the Lyme. My energy lever was regained and the mental fog was gone. I continued to get the Intravenous Vitamin C each week for a total of ten Vitamin C drips. My life returned to normal and I was very grateful. I started taking orally about five to ten grams of buffered Vitamin C almost every day for many years as a preventative, but after a while I thought taking this much Vitamin C was excessive so I cut down and eventually stopped taking Vitamin C to see how I would feel without supplemental Vitamin C. This was 1996 when I had the Vitamin C drips and the Vitamin C at that time was made from the Sago Palm Tree which I did not know at the time. Today most of the Vitamin C is now made from Genetically Modified Organisms, GMO corn and most of it comes from China. This Vitamin C from GMO corn is not as effective as the Sago Palm Vitamin C. I had gotten Lyme again many years later and the Doctor where I first went had stopped doing Intravenous Vitamin C drips. He recommended another facility and I went there and had a Vitamin C drip and it was not the same. I spoke to the Doctor there and I said, I do not think the Vitamin C is the same anymore and he said yes you are right. It is now being made from corn, but he said that his Vitamin C was made from camu camu which is a tropical fruit high in Vitamin C. I went for a few more Intravenous Vitamin C drips and some with some glutathione and some had the addition of a [Meyers Push which is an injection of some B vitamins, calcium and magnesium] but this was not working for me so I continued my journey for health and knew in my heart that there must be another way. I started calling vitamin companies and I have spoken with high end reputable vitamin companies about their products and if they are made using GMO products. One very popular, reputable vitamin company I spoke with told me when I asked if their Vitamin C and Vitamin E were made from GMOs, I was told they used GMO corn for Vitamin C and GMO soy for Vitamin E. I was told that when they are finished processing these vitamins made from GMO corn and GMO soy is that there is no detectable GMO material in the Vitamin C or Vitamin E. Vitamin companies are able to put on their vitamin label no GMOs because their tests detect no Genetically Modified Organisms GMOs even though these vitamins are made from GMO corn and GMO soy. I found another Vitamin C and the label said corn free. I emailed the company and asked what they made their corn free Vitamin C from and they emailed back from corn. I figured after processing their test did not know it was corn? From searching around I discovered that years ago Vitamin C was made from the Sago Palm Tree and that was what I had for my first Intravenous Vitamin C drip in 1996 and also Vitamin C supplements were made from the Sago Palm Tree at that time too. Astute health professionals of those days when Sago Palm Tree Vitamin C was prevalent, rave about how well Sago Palm

Tree Vitamin C worked. The Vitamin C from corn is not as effective as the Sago Palm Vitamin C. There is one company called Nutri-West that sells a Vitamin C pill supplement from Vitamin C made from the Sago Palm Tree that they said comes from China. Nutri-West mixes the Sago Palm Vitamin C with lemon bioflavonoids, rutin, hesperidin, and [thymus, lymph and spleen from bovine] and propolis. They told me the bovine material comes from grass fed cattle in Argentina. I have not taken this Vitamin C from Nutri-West because I did not want to take the glandulars thymus, lymph and spleen. There is another company called Pinnacle Laboritories that has a Vitamin C and the label says SAGO-C-Plus which I thought was made from the Sago Palm tree so I purchased some of the Vitamin C. I was thinking I should call the company and ask them what country they get the Sago Palm Tree Vitamin C. The person I spoke with said that their Vitamin C is no longer made from the Sago Palm Tree but now is made from corn even though the label still says Sago-C-

Plus. As Vitamin C made from corn became the main source for making Vitamin C, Twin Labs tried to keep making their Vitamin C from the Sago Palm Tree called Allergy C. On the front of the label of Allergy C it said corn free made from Sago Palm. I asked Twin Labs why they stopped making Vitamin C from the Sago Palm Tree and I was told, "Sago Palm is too expensive to compete with Vitamin C made from corn." It is too bad when people buy foods and supplements on price point along. Our body is the most expensive item we own. We need to maintain our body with the best. I get my Vitamin C from food and by having a slice of lemon or lime with meals and eat the skin too, the skin of lemons and limes are loaded with bioflavonoids. I also use Pure Synergy Pure Radiance C made from organic fruits. One rounded ¼ teaspoon is 180 mg of Vitamin C. Pure Synergy's Pure Radiance C from organic fruits and berries uses manioc root as the absorbent for the fruit and berry juice. If you see on a fruit and berry Vitamin C [malto-dextrin] which is used as an absorbent for the fruit and berry juice, then the malto-dextrin is most likely from GMO corn. Lemons and limes have enough Vitamin C to prevent scurvy and the lemon and lime skin is loaded with bioflavonoids. The 5th Century Chinese sailors used ginger to prevent scurvy. Though Intravenous Vitamin C was my first experience in relief from Lyme, I put this chapter near the end of the book. At first, I was not even going to write this chapter on Intravenous Vitamin C because of the lower quality of the Vitamin C made from GMO corn and I did not want to put religion in this book as it may offend some people. But as I was finishing this book I thought I should write a little bit about what I think is the most important article when it comes to health, and that is we should seek our Creator for the answers. In the Bible it says: Call to Me, and I will answer you, and show you great and mighty things, which you know not. Jeremiah chapter 33 verse 3. Our Creator knows what we need when man does not.

Chapter 34
Water

Hydrate, hydrate, hydrate. The body needs water. 50% to 60% of the body is water. Water is a river inside the body and acts as a delivery system for nutrients and removal of waste. Waste is removed through sweat, urine, bowel movements and respiration. I think it is a good practice to drink a glass of water a half to one hour before each meal. Drinking water before each meal gives a good kidney flush and hydrates the body to prepare for the meal to be eaten. We want to clear the kidneys with water before we eat a meal so the kidneys can filter waste products from eating, digesting and processing our meal. If we drink water during or after the meal we dilute the digestive enzymes in the gut putting a strain on the digestive system. It is best to hydrate and flush the kidneys before a meal. A rule of thumb on how much water to drink is half the body weight in [pounds] in ounces. Example if you weigh 100 pounds, 100 divided by 2 equals 50 ounces. Another rule of thumb for having sufficient water is the urine should be a light yellow. If the urine is dark yellow you need to drink more water. These are just guide lines to point us into the ball park and may not apply to everyone. The main thing is to drink enough water a half hour to one hour before a meal to get a good comfortable kidney flush [a pee in the toilet]. If you drink alcohol, do not think alcohol can replace water. Any drink that contains alcohol has some degree of dehydration and we must drink extra water to replace the dehydration degree of alcohol. Beer is the one alcoholic beverage that I think hydrates, though most beer has gluten and the gluten free beer in America at this time does not taste like beer. There are some very good gluten free beers in Europe that are made from low gluten barley and some of those beers go through a process that removes the gluten that I highly recommend if you like beer, though many people with Lyme are unable to drink alcohol without making their condition worse. After a person has been cleared of Lyme, moderate drinking of alcohol has many positive health benefits. If drinking of alcohol is excessive then alcohol becomes extremely counterproductive to good health and weakens the immune system and other systems and organs in the body. Get some good water. There is a website findaspring.com that has locations of springs around the world. If you do not have a local spring, an under the sink reverse osmosis with a post remineralizer may be a good option for you. Meat or fish with vegetables soup is also a great hydrator plus we get needed vitamins, minerals, electrolytes and amino acids from these soups too.

Chapter 35
Chiropractic For Better Health

Chiropractic is not just for back pain. Doing a once a week or once a month visit to the chiropractor has many benefits. If the spine is out of line [subluxated] it will affect the health of the body. Many people cannot feel that their spine is out of line because it can be a slow process that creeps up overtime and that person grows accustomed to being out of line ever so slowly and does not suspect anything. A person may say they feel just fine, but after starting chiropractic care they start to notice the overall improvements in their health. Not every chiropractor may be right for you. Find one you can trust. Finding a good chiropractic is worth more than their weight in gold. When I started chiropractic care I went to a chiropractor who looked to be about 250 to 300 pounds. When I was laying face down on the chiropractic table and this chiropractor adjusted my spine it felt like he was putting almost all 250 to 300 pounds on my back to adjust my spine. After this chiropractor adjusted me I felt like I had just finished a football game, actually worse. I figured that because I only weighed 130 pounds I could never be a chiropractor because of how hard this chiropractor had to push on my back to adjust my spine. Years later I was going to a chiropractor that is smaller than average man and he was able to adjust my spine with the slightest touch with hardly any pressure. I tell you this story so you can know it may take some time to find the right chiropractor for you. Backing up to the 250 to 300 pound chiropractor. One day I went in for an adjustment walking straight and after my adjustment I walked out the office walking with my back crooked to the side. I went looking for another chiropractor. Get some good recommendations from people you can trust. Take some time and find a good chiropractor it is worth it. Some chiropractors will adjust more than the spine, such as the thyroid, shoulder joints, knees and other joints too. Sometimes when someone gets a chiropractic adjustment there may be a little pain near the adjustment for a few days but this can be normal. Talk to your chiropractor and tell them about any pain and give them feedback positive or negative. This feedback will help the chiropractor with your care. If you do not like getting your spine manually adjusted look into Network Chiropractic also called Network Spinal Analysis. Network Spinal Analysis uses a gentle precise touch to the spine that cues the brain to create new wellness promoting strategies. These low force touches to the spine, assists the brain in developing new strategies to experience the world, adapt to stress, dissipate tension from the spine and nerves and connect with your body's natural rhythms. Network Chiropractic uses these low force touching points mostly on the back of the body, the chiropractors energy and your energy to induce the spine to adjust itself through your own body energy wave in the spine and connecting to the rest of the body. In Network Chiropractic the patient assists the chiropractor by relaxing as much as possible, allowing the releasing of trapped tension and allowing the body to correct itself. The Network chiropractor will sometimes tell you where to bring your attention in your body and to also sometimes breathe deeply. I cannot stress how important it is to find a good chiropractor. One may need to try many chiropractors before they find one that is a match for them.

Benefits of Chiropractic: Enhances immune system, promotes relaxation, improves digestive function, encourages cell regeneration, increases nutrient flow, reduces stiffness and pain, reduces recovery time, reduces muscle spasms, improves oxygenation, improves athletic performance.
Chiropractic Makes Life Better

Chapter 36
What Is Your Missing Nutrient

I do not eat corn, wheat or soybeans [except fermented soybeans in natto] and those ingredients are in chicken feed and what the chicken eats we eat too when we eat the chicken. I get my chickens for meat from a farmer who does not feed the chickens any corn, wheat or soybeans. I decided to get my own chickens for eggs and feed the chickens sunflower seeds, oats, hemp seeds, rice, plus green pasture and table scraps. I have since changed the diet of the chickens because I have found the eggs taste much better if the chickens are only feed sunflower seeds, hemp seeds, table scraps, some clabbered milk cheese and green pasture that has plenty of insects and worms. The yokes are orange and I could tell right away that the eggs were much more digestible for me and tasted better too. The breed of chicken I had at that time did not lay eggs in the cold winter, which I did not know when I first got the chickens. Winter came and the chickens stopped laying eggs. I would look in different stores for eggs that were feed similar to how I fed my chickens. In one store I found some duck eggs that said on the label, no corn, no wheat and no soy. Excited I bought some duck eggs and when I cooked them they tasted great. The duck eggs were more digestible for me that regular organic grain fed chicken eggs but not as digestible as my home flock chicken eggs. I emailed the duck farmer to ask what they feed their ducks. The farmer emailed back and said their ducks are fantastic grazers and eat mostly grass and a mix that they make of barley, spelt and sunflower seeds. Barley and spelt have gluten and that is why I noticed the duck eggs were not as digestible as my chicken eggs, but I liked the taste of the duck eggs so much and read that duck eggs are more nutritious than chicken eggs. I decided to get my own ducks in the spring so I could feed them the same way I feed my chickens. When I got the baby ducks I put them in a stock tank with bedding food and water. I fed them rice, ground up sunflower seeds, oats and greens. For the first week they were active, growing, content and happy to see me when I brought food and water. The second week they became lethargic, afraid and some of the ducks were not walking very well. I immediately looked up to see if I could find any information on ducks and leg problems. I found that baby ducks require more niacin during their first two months of life than is usually found in chicken feed and if they do not get enough niacin they can develop leg problems. I read that ducks on pasture find enough insects and worms to get their necessary niacin but these ducks were too young to put out on pasture without a mother duck. I immediately ordered some liquid niacin and found the right amount to add in their water. I had some dried insects and gave them to the ducks to eat hoping this would help and they did eat a lot of the dried insects but the next day one duck could not walk at all and both legs were flared out to each side and her head down with eyes closed and I thought she might die because she was so weak and incoherent. I put this duck in a separate box by herself to give her the care she may need. I mixed up some niacin in water and took a dropper full of niacin water and put some in the duck's mouth because she did not have the strength to drink herself as her eyes were closed and her neck limp and she looked like she would die. I picked up some organic grower chicken feed and started giving it to the other ducks along with niacin in their water too. I gave this duck as much of the niacin water from the dropper as I thought she could take that day. The next day this ducks eyes were open and she was able to lift her head a little and was receptive to me giving her more niacin water from a dropper but still too weak to eat any chicken feed. It was about the fourth day that this duck was showing more sign of progress and was able to drink some niacin water for herself and eat some chicken feed. She still could not walk or even stand up so I put the niacin water and chicken feed right next to her. One bowl on each side and she was able to drink and eat herself. I had to clean her bedding every day. It was amazing to see how one nutrient in water for a few days without any food was able to start a turn around with this duck that was at deaths door. Each day this duck that could not walk improved. She started being able to wiggle herself around the box she was in and showing more strength. I would then take this duck out of her private box and put her in the stock tank with the other ducks for the night. The other ducks at night would surround this duck and lay their necks on her neck. It was quite a display of affection. In the morning I would take the duck that could not walk out of the stock tank because she could not stand up and reach the food and niacin water in the stock tank with the other ducks. She needed her food on the ground in order to eat and drink and if I put her food on the ground in the stock tank with the other ducks they could walk in her food and water making it unclean with manure. When I would take the duck that could not walk out of the stock tank in the morning to her own box she would scream at me no no no in duck language. Each day this duck got stronger and stronger and then one day one of her legs started to propel her around her box but the other was limp. Every night she got to sleep with her siblings and during the day she went to her own box for special care. I then thought I should put her in a small bowl of warm water, not too deep but where she would float and her legs would hang down and be able to still touch the bottom of the bowl and maybe she could move her legs easily through the water and this would be good rehabilitation. I put her in the warm water and it did not take but a few seconds for her to start moving her legs and ducking her head under the water and I could see she was loving it. I continued with this rehabilitation each day and each day she grew stronger and the leg that was limp became stronger too. This duck could not walk yet but she became able to stand for a few seconds. As time went by this duck got stronger and stronger and started taking a few steps now and then until one day she could walk, and after about two months looked like she never had a problem. The other ducks recovered much quicker and the whole flock turned out to be good egg laying happy ducks. I was so amazed and impressed by how one nutrient could make such a difference between life and death for these ducks. It made me think "what is my missing nutrient or nutrients." I wanted to share this event I witnessed with my eyes with you, to have you think what may be your missing nutrient or nutrients.

I hope the information in this book will help you on your journey to abundant health. Blessings! Tom Pote

Appendix

Tickcheck.com
If bitten by a tick. Tickcheck.com can determine if the tick carries Lyme or other tick-borne diseases.
Book recommendations:
Iodine Why You Need It Why You Can't Live Without It By David Brownstein M.D.
The Iodine Crisis What You Don't Know About Iodine Can Wreck Your Life' By Lynne Farrow.
Lick The Sugar Habit: Sugar Addiction Upsets Your Whole Body Chemistry by Nancy Appleton
The Case Against Sugar By Gary Taubes
A Consumer's Dictionary of Food Additives by Ruth Winter M.S.
Food Additives: A Shoppers Guide to What's Safe & What's Not!
By Christine Hoza Farlow D.C.
The Whole Soy Story: The Dark Side of America's Favorite Health Food
By Kaayla Daniels
Devil In The Milk: Illness, Health and Politics of A1 and A2 Milk
By Keith Woodford and Thomas Cowan
Nutrition and Physical Degeneration
by Weston A. Price

www.ingramcontent.com/pod-product-compliance
Lightning Source LLC
Chambersburg PA
CBHW070529220526
45467CB00003B/920